HELP YOURSELF!

The Bircher-Benner clinic of Zurich, Switzerland, specializes in the nutritional treatment of disease. Its staff of physicians has developed an internationally acclaimed program of meal planning, treatment, and physical fitness that is outlined in a series of outstanding health guides.

The Arthritis and Rheumatism Nutrition Plan has everything you need to know about rheumatism and their treatment, including:

- Comprehensive physical and medical treatment for these diseases.

- How to guard against the recurrence of arthritis and rheumatism.

- Common viruses, infections and dental problems that can lead to arthritis.

- How to help treat arthritis and rheumatism with diet.

ABOUT THE
BIRCHER-BENNER CLINIC

In the nineteenth century, Dr. M. Bircher-Benner wanted to established a kind of clinic that had never existed before: a clinic that would take into account the whole man, both body and soul, not only the patient's disease; a clinic that would use an intelligent patient as a co-worker in a total therapeutic effort; a clinic that would use the total knowledge of modern medicine to support the "internal physician"—the autonomous healing forces and healing system of the body—and in every case make the healing effects of dietetic therapy and one's life-style the basis of a total health plan; a clinic that, in addition to eliminating immediate ailments, would bring about a new, tougher, more satisfying and creative health of body and soul for the patient.

The private clinic founded by Dr. Bircher-Benner in 1897 is still operated today for that purpose.

Bircher - Benner Nutrition Plan for Arthritis and Rheumatism

A Comprehensive Guide With Suggestions for Diet Menus and Recipes

Translated by Lotte Erlich

By the staff of the Bircher-Benner Clinic:

Medical/Dietetic Section:
*D. Liechti-v. Brasch,
M.D., P. F. Boesch, M.D.,
S. Grieder-Dopheide, M.D.*

Physiological/Chemical Section:
Alfred Kunz-Bircher, Ph.D.

Menus and Recipes:
*Ruth Kunz-Bircher, M.D.
(head of the Bircher-Benner Clinic)*

Edited by *Ralph Bircher, M.D.*

PYRAMID BOOKS NEW YORK

BIRCHER-BENNER NUTRITION PLAN FOR
ARTHRITIS AND RHEUMATISM

A PYRAMID BOOK

Copyright © 1972 by Nash Publishing

Pyramid edition published October 1976

ISBN: 0-515-4224-2

Library of Congress Catalog Card Number: 70-186901

Pyramid Books are published by Pyramid Publications (Harcourt Brace
Jovanovich, Inc.). Its trademarks, consisting of the word "Pyramid"
and the portrayal of a pyramid, are registered in the United States
Patent Office.

PYRAMID PUBLICATIONS (Harcourt Brace Jovanovich, Inc.).
757 Third Avenue, New York, N.Y. 10017

Contents

I. Introduction

To Be Read Carefully By Every Rheumatic Patient

Chronic rheumatic inflammation of the joints is generally not a dramatic and, certainly, not a fatal disease, and for this reason, has been relatively neglected by medical research for a long time. Yet it has caused the human race greater distress than many a deadly disease, and to those concerned and for those around them it is often an exceedingly painful and prolonged affliction. For the invalidism of arthritis can last a long time: on the average it permits its victims to survive for about twenty years (Belart).

Let a healthy person envision for a brief moment the fate of one who has been struck by the full impact of this disease: However bravely he may have stood up to the vicissitudes of life, studied and worked, proved himself and attained a respected position—none of it is of much help to him now. Unmercifully, the disease overwhelms him with violent pain, limits his movements, and leaves him unable to work. Just now, in the prime of life, when he might enjoy the fruits of his labor, by rights could and should be a support, guardian, experienced adviser and fount of knowledge to his family, his colleagues, to the younger generation, at that precise moment he is rendered a helpless wreck. He has to let everything go, he is confined to a wheelchair or even lying stretched out on his bed, a helpless bundle wracked by pain—"a burden unto himself and to others, and not good for anything any more," as one of these unfortunates expressed it.

7

What is Rheumatism?

"Rheuma" stems from the Greek term meaning to "flow" and describes the painful disease of connective tissues, joints, muscles, their inflammation with or without fever, acute or chronic, singularly affecting joints then passing away and afflicting other joints. In an acute case, the patient will suffer from severe pain, occasionally with high temperatures and serious immobility. In primary and secondary rheumatic cases, pains will be mild, but joints will gradually feel more stiff, deformed, and may eventually lead to total invalidism.

"Arthritis" stands for the inflammation of the joints; "polyarthritis" (or PA) for the inflammation of a great number of joints.

1. Acute and Chronic Polyarthritis (PA)

An acute condition may turn into a chronic state and is then called "secondary chronic PA." Its causes usually are infections, toxics, and allergies. Infections may stem from tonsils, teeth, jaw, and sinus, intestines (appendix, colon), gall bladder, renal pelvis, etc. It may also stem from acute virus illnesses such as scarlet fever, typhus, viral hepatitis. It is known, however, that these infections only lead to polyarthritis if the body is unusually receptive to it, i.e. where mesenchyme (network of tissues giving rise to connective tissue, blood lymphatics, bone, and cartilage), metabolism, and hormonal glands act as a breeding ground. Thus, poorly balanced nutrition with a disturbance in the proportions of acid and alkaline nutrients cannot act as a defense against such infections and allergies, but will aid any rheumatic tendencies.

Overeating, with meals too heavy in denatured carbohydrates, animal protein, and fats, a lack of raw vegetables and fruits (particularly a lack in vitamins C, B and E) will further create an ideal climate for rheumatics. In addition, most people lack physical exercise outdoors through which the body attunes itself to climatic changes, humidity, cold and warm weather spells. Any weather change will be a burden to the untrained who is quick to blame the "bad weather" for his rheumatism. A healthy, well-nourished, and physically trained body can stand such climatic changes.

Further, excessive, prolonged stress, deep psychological shock, and depression may also lead to polyarthritis. This was particularly evident during the war when hunger, cold, and fear prevailed. It may also occur in women after childbirth, as ovarian functions play an important role in rheumatic development. It is interesting to note that women may be free of rheumatism entirely during pregnancy due to an abundance of hormones, but may experience relapses after giving birth. Some people with rheumatism were, at one time, experimentally given blood transfusions from pregnant women, and further deterioration was brought to a halt. Underfunctioning of the ovaries and menstrual disorders are often connected with PA and must thus be considered when treating rheumatism.

The adrenal gland, in particular, is exposed to all kinds of stress and is not strong enough to withstand it for a prolonged period of time. It regulates with other glands, the energy reserves of the body and acts as a reservoir for vitamin C. Its failure to function will provoke PA. Once the importance of the adrenal gland's defense mechanism was recognized, treatment with the adrenal-gland hormone, cortisone, was introduced and later superseded by prednisone; thus a new era in treatment of rheumatism had begun.

Through research and experience, physicians have time and again seen demonstrated that complete recovery, without side effects and free of danger, can only be achieved if treatment is based on a rejuvenation of the metabolism and whole body, both in physical and emotional terms, to make it more effective in the fight against viruses and allergies. In the case of rheumatic polyarthritis, one must distinguish between acute, primary, and secondary chronic types.

2. Arthrosis

This is a non-inflammatory degeneration which occurs with advanced age, primarily in women after menopause, but also in men. The patient suffers from pain and swelling of the joints, which are, however, not inflamed, nor does he experience any fever or reddening. The joints literally "dry out," the cartilage layers become thinner and dryer, bones lose calcium (osteoporosis) and the joints gradually begin to feel stiffer. The spine's vertebrae are frequently attacked, causing them to bulge, and the back gradually begins to feel stiffer and less mobile (spondylarthrosis). The hip joints, should they be involved, lose their round form and become painful when walking or moving around (coxarthrosis). Knuckles become thick and pressure-sensitive. Most often, knees are affected particularly in cases of obesity (gonarthrosis). Many decades of the aging process have prepared for this hormonal regression, and general metabolic condition. It will pay you to heed and deal with this. Detoxifying and balanced nourishment, ridding the body of excess fluid, provides a regulatory groundwork, and should be supported by physical therapy such as mineral baths, physiotherapy and massages. Control of hormones is particularly important for women.

3. Arthritis of Gout (arthritis uratica)

An unprecedented increase of gout has been taking place recently. This disease is often mistaken for rheumatism. It forms an entirely different image and is caused by an imbalance of uric acid and its deposits of crystals in the ball of a joint, bone, and cartilage. It is usually hereditary, but a diet free of uric acid can play an important part in the treatment of this form of arthritis and can serve in the prevention of further complications such as gouty kidney and gouty liver. Gout is the "sickness of Kings" (Henry VIII); it is called the disease of a too-sophisticated society, and it usually disappears in wartime.

Causes and Treatment of Rheumatic Illnesses

According to statistics, 7½-8 percent of the total population suffers from chronic rheumatism, and most of these in what we call primary rheumatic stage upon which we will concentrate in this book. For the U.S., this means 16-17 million people and a yearly increase of rheumatic/ arthritic invalids of more than one million—many more than are caused by traffic accidents.

Exhaustive research reveals that a deterioration of the soft connective tissue which surrounds the joint bones (head and socket) and the muscles, in its less severe forms, can be found in 97% of all persons over sixty years of age. The deterioration consists of a roughening of the tissue, thus impeding the gliding motion of the bone head in its socket.

After all this, the reader will not be surprised to learn about the following momentous sentence contained in the introduction to a proposal for a Swiss law for the fight against rheumatism: "From a social and economic point of view, rheumatism is probably *the most serious* disease afflicting the population." In fact the annual cost imposed by rheumatic diseases on the economy is estimated at 400 million francs for Switzerland and 220 million pound sterling for Great Britain (roughly in U.S. dollars, respectively 99.4 million and 670 million).

In view of this situation, it is easy to understand that, at present, every conceivable effort is directed to research in the prevention, treatment, and care in this field. In fact, such efforts have recently multiplied. Research into rheumatism has developed strongly, and excellent centers have been set up, such as that of the Rheuma-Liga in Switzerland. This is a comfort for the afflicted and creates much highly welcomed relief for suffering. Yet, the main task remains: to prevent and heal this disease. Although many new and more effective medications have been added to the traditional ones in the last few years, all of them only act to check the inflammation and reduce the pain and remain effective only as long as they are taken. Indeed, they are momentarily welcome and capable of causing temporary relief in cases of need, as an expert (Belart) sums up the situation; but their continuous use is not without danger. More or less severe damage can result, and thus improvements are often treacherous. Serious complications can also arise when medication is interrupted. Inflammations and even pain, by their very nature, are an expression of the organism's efforts at resistance and healing. One does not help these efforts at self-healing by suppression; on the contrary, one hinders the exact process which might possibly lead to a cure. The disease, in its chronic course, is not overcome by these remedies, frequently it is even aggravated. For this reason, it is specific to many treatments directed primarily toward relief that the suffering, after interruption of the treatment, reemerges anew in its old intensity, and that the remedies become less effective each time, until finally the disease takes its predestined course. The newly developed medications have a sharply limited scope: their action can bridge an acute condition until a more purposeful and basic treatment can take effect.

Considering the depressing character of the disease it is all too easy to understand that, in spite of everything, new hope is raised again and again by every new medication. This was already so after 1876, when *salicylic acid* (present in aspirin) was introduced in the treatment of rheumatic diseases, a medication which, in spite of all the newer, more powerful remedies, to this day plays the principal part in the treatment of rheumatism, because it is relatively safe. It was thought that in salicylic acid a genuine remedy had been discovered; and yet, it had to be recognized that its only effect has been to suppress the swelling and thus to relieve the pain, and that it has no effect on the disease itself. Recently, even the relative safety of this medication has been questioned. It was found that it does have poisonous side effects which are easily overlooked, and that tolerance to it varies according to the individual.

Thus it was established that many undiagnosed stomach hemorrhages and anemias had to be attributed to treatment with salicylic acid. Blood loss was found in 70% of patients treated with aspirin (according to Stubbe). Salicylic acid is particularly dangerous when hidden inflammations or ulcers in the digestive tract are present. Other, newer rheumatism remedies may also trigger or aggravate such ulcers. Unfortunately, the apparent safety of the salicylic-acid treatment has for a considerable time led to its uncritical use, even for children. It soon became apparent that children are the most endangered because with them the leeway between the therapeutic dosage (30-35 mg%) and the toxic dosage (30-59 mg%) is particularly small. The most serious objection against protracted treatment with salicylic acid is probably the fact that this remedy appears eventually to damage the soft connective tissue (mesenchyme) and thus diminishes the prospects of a genuine cure (Bovet).

Gold therapy still plays a certain part in the treatment of arthritis today, and in certain cases it achieves greater relief than salicylic acid. However the leeway between the therapeutic dosage and the toxic dosage is very narrow, and, in addition, there are great fluctuations from person to person, so that it can only be applied with great care and experience and under strict controls. As far as possible we avoid gold therapy completely, because it may interfere with the efficacy of the physical-dietetic therapy applied at the same time.

In 1949 *hormone* treatment of arthritis with *cortisone* and *ACTH* was discovered. A film of the Mayo Clinic in the U.S.A. showed successful cures, such as had never been seen before, in patients with chronically inflamed joints after a few injections. Who cannot remember the wave of hope which then swept over the world? Leading publications such as *Life* and *Time* wrote at the time: "The new therapy is likely to alter the horrible countenance of the manifestations of arthritic disease. The discovery will probably become a milestone in the history of medicine." For among all the diseases afflicting mankind, arthritis has the most crippling effect on body and mind, and it affects more people than tuberculosis, polio, and cancer together. Until a short time before, nobody had even an inkling on how to heal this disease. In its long and desperate search, medicine had explored all possible avenues . . . "but none of these treatments," continues the article, "is in any sense a way to a permanent cure." Their largest value is "that they make the patient feel that something is being done for him." Some treatments seem to provide beneficial results, but only temporarily. And all this would be changed by the newly developed hormone treatment, so it was believed at that time, and a genuine cure for arthritis would be at hand.

The dangers of one-sided and routine hormone treatments have since been recognized, and are the reasons that science is searching today for ways of clearly elucidating the value of a more specific and individually applied hormone treatment as a temporary support for a natural therapy. The action of the newest preparations in this field—prednisone, hydrocortisone and others—is just as temporary as that of the other preparations, and, because of possible side effects, they must be used with care in a limited way. Their greatest drawback is that they weaken the activity of the ductless glands—the pituitary, adrenals, thyroid, pancreas, etc.—and can cause their stunting, even where the more serious side effects are avoided through careful dosage.

In spite of all the uncertainty concerning the causes of chronic rheumatic inflammations of the joints, we definitely know today that at the basis of the disease is a *degeneration of the soft connective tissue* (mesenchyme) in the whole body, as Belart has stated in his survey of the situation. This mesenchyme, comparable to a fine layer of foam rubber, permeates the entire body and surrounds all the organs and the blood vessels with a cushioning, especially the heads and sockets of the joint bones. For this reason, a truly curative therapy of rheumatism and rheumatoid arthritis must above all be directed toward the task of overcoming the degeneration of this soft connective tissue which leads to these diseases. The clinician, Dr. Sihle (*Über das Weltbild des Arztes und den Sinn der Krankheit*) compares the mesenchyme to a flowerbed. For it is actually much more than the mere cushion which it had been considered to be for a long time; it is the breeding ground on which the organs prosper or pine away, according to what condition it is in. Much research has been expended on the rehabilitation of this breeding ground, the mesenchyme, and many have vainly attempted to solve this problem in a variety of ways. So far the most successful has been the Eppinger-School at the Vienna University Clinic. These researchers and clinicians explored all avenues to find the causes of the frequently occurring edema and diffuse thickening of this connective tissue, in order to heal this abnormality. Were they successful, they calculated, the drama "Disease" in general, and of any type whatsoever, would have been diminished somewhat in the first act, and, from the healed breeding ground, healing processes must then come forth with many remedial results, just as, earlier, sickness had arisen from the degenerated mesenchyme. The results of all these experiments were not conclusive until a (salt-free) treatment with raw fruit was instituted exactly according to. Dr. Bircher-Benner's directions. When treatment was started early enough, an unequivocal and lasting recovery and revitalization of the soft connective tissues of the entire body of the patient could be observed; and simultaneously, when this happened, the cells of the organism gained the ability of selecting from among the nutrients presented it— a sure sign of tissue recovery—and the defensive and self-healing mechanisms of the organs increased in force and intensity (Prof. Hans Eppinger, M.D., "Über Rohkostbehandlung," *Wiener Klinische Wochenschrift 5/26-38*).

Thus, in a diet of raw natural food ("raw diet"), as it has been tried and developed for many decades in the Bircher-Benner Clinic (and elsewhere), lies the possibility of overcoming the rheumatic constitution by treating one of its causes, namely the degeneration of the mesenchyme. This diet constitutes the *basic treatment* to be applied in every case, and it can be supported by many valuable procedures to regulate and revitalize the mesenchyme and restore the body's mobility.

The condition of the soft connective tissues affects the most varied bodily systems. This is especially the case when, through generations, a human type has evolved which is prone to rheumatic diseases: asthenic-leptosomatic body build, dominance of the vagotonic nervous system, poor circulation, anemia, irregularities at puberty, psychosomatic misdirection, lack of control, and abnormal intestinal conditions. These various malfunctions tend to interact and be dependent upon each other. Thus, long experience reveals that, under the influence of diet, distinct changes can be seen in the microscopic picture of the capillaries of such patients as well as a reversal in the formation of blood sludge.

Arthritis appears to have an additional "breeding ground" which, in a way, serves to protect the mesenchyme: the *digestive system*. According to our experience, sufferers from arthritis always evidence more or less extensive deterioration of the intestinal bacterial flora and a weakening of the defensive functions of the intestinal walls. Here we have a further possibility of influencing arthritis through a suitable curative diet via the intestinal tract! A further therapeutic effect of the natural diet is that it creates the conditions and the correct inner climate for a healthy intestinal bacterial flora by its own particular richness in enzymes. It was previously believed that the (highly sensitive) enzymes of the living plant cells could not survive passage through the intestinal tract. But, somehow, in a way not yet discovered, they are protected from destruction, and it can be proved that 60-80 percent of them reach the large intestine (Tropp and Chalaupka) and there fulfill their important function: This consists in their combining with the oxygen available and thus providing the anaerobic (oxygen-free) climate necessary for a healthy intestinal flora. To the extent that intestinal bacteria capable of regeneration are still present, it is possible for the intestinal flora to recover on its own, on a predominantly natural diet. Otherwise it is possible to help it along in various ways (Bioghurt, Ribolac, Colivakzine, etc.).

Since under the influence of this diet, the desired changes occur in the intestinal area and digestive functions, even long-standing constipation with chronic decay and fermentation can be overcome. Thus, digestion becomes not only trouble-free, but utilization of the nutrients is also greatly improved and deficiencies are overcome. The result is a significant relief from stress and a detoxification of many organs, the whole organism, and, above all, also of the soft connective tissues.

II. The Experiment at the Royal Free Hospital in London Using the Restorative Diet in Rheumatoid Arthritis

It is difficult for a contemporary, expert or not, to believe that anything as simple and natural as fresh raw fruit, raw vegetables, and nuts are capable of causing significant bodily reactions, and especially that with the help of those reactions the cure of severe rheumatic inflammation of the joints of long standing should be possible, without the use of the latest achievements of pharmaceutical science. Therefore we shall cite here the successful results obtained by expert utilization of the healing action of plant substances and properties in the following experiment, carried out at the Royal Free Hospital in London, England, in order to record the curative effect of Dr. Bircher-Benner's natural fresh-food diet (in a documentary film*).

This experiment came about in the following way: One day the London Hospital was confronted with the problem of treating an extreme case of chronic rheumatic inflammation of the joints such as are frequently encountered in the rheumatism section of the hospital. The patient was utterly helpless and had been prostrate on her bed for some time, barely capable of any activity other than scant and painful movements of the extremities. It was beyond all reasonable medical expectation to attain even palliative help with known medical measures. The demands of care

---

* The report on the results of this experiment may be found in the Proceedings of the Royal Society of Medicine Vol. XXX, London, England.

were excessive. At the suggestion of one of the attending physicians the patient was transferred to Zurich and was cured by the dietetic-physical therapy at the Bircher-Benner Clinic. After several months the patient was able to return home by train. The physicians in London confirmed the cure and were sufficiently unprejudiced to look into the matter. They sent a woman doctor to Zurich who thoroughly investigated and studied the entire treatment on the spot. After her return to London she reported on what she had seen and was then assigned a twenty-bed ward for this type of treatment of arthritic patients. As soon as the first positive results were observed in the section it was decided to film the course of the successful treatment in a number of patients. Arthritis presents a technologically favorable picture for filming because it attacks the joints, affecting the freedom of movement. It is easy to represent on film the changes and the painfulness in the patient's ability to move. In severe cases the changes in the bones and cartilage can be recorded by X-ray.

With a view to getting clear-cut results, the cases selected were treated by diet alone, strictly according to the Zurich diet directions: beginning with two weeks of a raw diet only and followed by the gradual addition of whole cereals, steamed vegetables, potatoes boiled in their skins, and vegetable bouillon. All palliative treatments, especially drugs, were omitted. The cases selected for the test were twelve patients who were judged incurable and were suffering from acute primary and secondary chronic arthritis. The result was as follows: Seven complete, three partial recovery of mobility, and two, no improvement at all. All twelve patients showed considerable improvement in their general condition at the end of the treatment . . . The most remarkable among these twelve cases was the tenth. At the end of treatment this case had made the least progress toward full mobility. At the beginning of treatment, this female patient was 55 years old, had been suffering from secondary chronic polyarthritis in its fifth stage for years, and for the last six weeks she had been in a condition very similar to that of the patient who had been sent to Zurich: crippled fingers, stiff joints with distinct roentgenologic changes, stiff spine, inability to sit up or remain sitting, emaciation from lack of exercise. All she could do was lift her arms and legs a little, and she was dependent on other persons for all needs.

The film then shows this patient first with her limited capacity for movement, prone and emaciated, and an X-ray of the changes in her joints. Then she is shown at various stages of the treatment, where she is executing certain specific movements for comparison of progress. At the start, the patient appears to be beyond all hope of recovery. Even after six weeks—two weeks of strict and four weeks of the less strict diet—progress is hardly worth mentioning, so that the attending physicians are ready to give up hope. The patient is now able to sit up for short periods, and the pain is less severe. Mobility is still minimal. But the patient herself now wants to continue. She has a feeling that "it is coming," that the process of self-healing has intensified . . . April 1st. The patient can be helped to sit and can bear to sit up for a short while. At the same time she exercises her knee and ankle joints.

. . . On the fifth of May, attempts to walk can be started in a walker.

. . . June 27th. Begins walking exercise with the help of crutches.

This perseverance pays off. But first there is a test for the patient, because she has an apparent "relapse." Fever and pain increase instead of decreasing. This is one of those critical phases in every cure which is triggered by the reactivation of the natural self-healing processes of the organism. Frequently the fever and pain are indications that the organism is fighting for recovery as it has not done for a long time. To the fainthearted and uninformed it looks like a worsening of the condition. Fears and doubts arise, and the relatives worry and urge that the treatment be stopped. In such phases of the treatment everything depends on the courage and perseverance of the physician and his patient which, in this case, was outstanding. Both of them struggled courageously and persistently for a successful cure. The patient persevered even during the hardest phase, which occurred in the seventh week.

Now we observe an increase in mobility . . . At first the patient attempts to walk, suspended in a walker, then supported by crutches, slowly, step by step, setting one foot in front of the other (she has to relearn to walk from the beginning); then with the help of two canes, later with one cane, becoming constantly somewhat more mobile. The sole treatment still consists of the raw diet with supplements, and encouragement increases with progress, which, though time-consuming, yet appears incredible. But the patient has to continue to be patient, and all participants need patience, too. The uphill course is steady, but slow. The recovery of keeping balance while walking takes longest. This needs to be painfully relearned. The bone and cartilage of the joints are completely changed and can regain its original shape only in part, if at all. It is fortunate that the human organism has such great adaptability, sometimes almost bordering on the miraculous. Thanks to this, the patient even here is eventually capable of lifting her arms and bending from the hips to touch her toes without falling over, and finally can move along without the use of cane or support.

After a little more than a year, the patient is able to return to her family. She is now capable of doing light housework chores and can help herself. This is the partial recovery of mobility which is mentioned in the final report as one of the three partial successes. The mobility of a normal, healthy person of the same age has unfortunately not been reached by a long way, but to the patient it is a blessing, and to those about her it is a "miracle."

. . . Two weeks later (December 2) she walks slowly without a cane, led only by the hand and rises from her chair by herself.

. . . One year after admission (February 20) a deep bend in proof of recovery of full hip mobility . . . Discharged on April 20.

How will the patient progress at home? Will she be able to retain the level of mobility attained, or will she slide back into her previous condition?

It was ten years later that we heard again about this patient. Once when the film was shown to English guests, there was a young woman among them who, at the moment the arthritis patient appeared on the screen in her prostrated early condition, exclaimed: "Why—that's my mother!" From her we got further information, not only about her history, but also about her later course. Above all, we were told how she was now, ten years later, and that was the most amazing part: According to the daughter she was now, at the age of 66, able to work for two hours in succession in the garden and to dig with a spade! On a diet which, on medical advice, had been much less strict and subject to many deviations and exceptions during visits and on festive occasions, there was yet at home a steady progress in recovery with no relapses. The exceptions and deviations were tolerated without ill effects, once the patient had reached a certain level of capacity to heal herself. However, will a patient not become completely emaciated and enfeebled on a diet consisting to four fifths of raw vegetables and fruit, and which supplies almost exclusively vegetable proteins— at a time when he should finally regain his strength and put on some weight? According to all dietetic rules, would this not be the time when the diet ought to be enriched with animal protein? In actual fact the film demonstrates that just this scanty, predominantly vegetarian diet rebuilds a body which, for an almost 56-year-old person, is full and harmoniously shaped, and that the patient's strength increases. The diet has restored to the organism what in our opinion has to be considered as of prime importance for a cure and recovery of strength: *economy in the metabolism.* The organism, which previously had resisted all attempts to build it up with "nourishing" food, can once again fully utilize the proffered nourishment, with little strain on the digestive system; it is able to "make a little go a long way" instead of "making little out of plenty!"

This case, together with the other eleven cases in the experiment at the Royal Free Hospital, do not yet constitute extensive statistics for recovery. The significance of the film lies predominantly in the unequivocal demonstration of the results achieved by the sole application of this diet by way of strengthening the self-curative forces and the autonomous recovery processes, which, if properly supported, do endeavor to restore wholesome order in the organism as far as possible.

Unfortunately the disease is sometimes so advanced and severely chronic that the patient is too far gone and incurable. Degenerative conditions exist where the self-healing processes of the body have lost their power. This is, for example, the case, where complete stiffening of the bones has occurred. The prognosis for this type of case is unfortunately today frequently even less favorable than after the war, if for a long time only intensive medical treatment has been given and valuable time has been lost for the application of natural, unspecific therapeutic factors. In addition, in such severe cases treatment places extraordinary demands on the patient and nursing personnel. In most cases, chronically ill polyarthritis patients suffer from depression. They have often given up any hope for recovery and lost their will power to start a new healing process. Any relapses, which have to be considered, as described herein, cannot be overcome because of lack of persistence. The physician is then required to assist the patient not only with his medical knowledge but also through positive encouragement and will to reach the goal.

On the other hand, a specialized medical establishment does by no means only use diet, as was the case in the Royal Free Hospital experiment, but the curative effect, as previously indicated, is supported and advanced by many other valuable means. In the treatment of a rheumatic, physiotherapy in conjunction with a raw food diet, is indispensable.

It will now be understood how extremely important it is to make people understand the need for early, comprehensive action. One cannot expect any quick improvement, not through natural physical-dietetic, nor, where necessary, through additional medical treatment, when the regulatory and glandular systems of the organism have been malfunctioning for years. One has to persevere patiently and consistently for months or even years if one still wants to attain one's goals. If gold or extended prednisone treatments have been prescribed, the healing process is further complicated.

As a counterpart, let us briefly mention another case, in

which an intelligent female patient applied the curative diet at the very moment when it still had the best prospects of success.

The patient was living in the environs of Zurich, she was also a 55-year-old teacher, still active in her profession, but now afraid she might have to retire prematurely. Due to the arthritis in the joints of her knees she could hardly get to her school any more. The idea of having to give up her beloved profession depressed her greatly. After seeing the film of the Royal Free Hospital, she followed the instructions as they are given in this booklet, at home, determined to let nothing stand in her way as far as was in her power. In a few weeks she recovered from the rheumatic inflammation of her knee joints, so that for the following ten years she was able to practice her profession without impediment until she reached the legal retirement age. She is still active and enterprising even today. Relapses occurred in the inflammation of her knee joints under unusual stress or after festivities with excessive dietary indulgence. However a short period of dieting would quickly eliminate the distress.

The arthritis film of the Royal Free Hospital makes one wonder why a therapy of such obvious efficacy has not found much wider acceptance. This diet treatment has indeed been tried and has proved its value in a number of hospitals and sanatoria in several countries; but this was only possible when one did not merely rely on recipes and directions, but took the trouble to prepare the food in the proper composition and manner, and where the time factor was duly taken into account. Where these conditions are not considered, the danger of failure is great. But if provisions are to be made in this respect, then the administration of the institution and the manager of the private household must be in full support of the project, the kitchen staff has to be trained, and utensils have to be bought. As is well known, kitchens are often run according to firmly established ideas and principles, and it can easily happen that— without ill will—the staff will quietly modify suggested procedures, if the attending physician does not take the trouble of frequently tasting the food and of convincing himself personally that the correct procedures are being followed, even taking a hand himself and demonstrating them, if necessary. For this reason it is also essential that the reader study this manual with care and that he refer back to it again and again. The diet has to be tasty and agreeable to the eye. It has to offer variety if it is to be followed for any length of time. Gradually, the patient will then come to like the therapeutic diet and learn to value it. The concepts of taste change, and new qualities are discovered in the food.

To the patient, this diet is usually something entirely new, to which he is unaccustomed. He is burdened with the prejudices of his surroundings. Thus, the attending physician or the dietician must spare no effort to explain the meaning, the principle, and the mode of action of the diet over and over, to alleviate the common fear of undernourishment which is apt to lead to senseless overeating, and patiently to teach slow and careful chewing. The only way to achieve all this is probably to sit occasionally at the table with the patient, to watch him, and to encourage him.

Relatives, nurses, and doctors should not depreciate the therapy by their actions or by their remarks, something which often happens from sheer ignorance. Encouragement helps! Gradually confidence in one's own strength grows, and with it inner independence of outside opinion. Every once in a while that popular devil "idle talk" lurks around a corner. In the critical phases or therapeutic crises which were mentioned above, the patient's self confidence and trust is often sorely tried. Taking all this into consideration, one can easily understand that, in order to persevere, the patient needs some measure of independence, maturity, and intelligence. But every small advance he makes in self-control and perseverance will fill him with satisfaction, growing confidence, and joy, and be of benefit to him throughout his lifetime.

If one considers these basic presumptions, one can easily understand that, however motivated the physician may be to help the arthritic patient, it is not easy for him to follow this path, although it presents such incomparably better prospects of a cure than any other. For these very reasons, doctors and patients wishing to use the therapeutic diet need, as has become obvious over and over, a practical help of a particular kind to achieve their ends, namely, such a manual as is presented here. Its purpose is to simplify the instructions for the physician, and to provide the patient and his entourage with the explanations, instructions, and aids, necessary to enable them to carry through a cure which often requires planning ahead for a considerable time.

III. Treatment

The patient's physical and emotional balance has usually been more or less affected by his painful condition and the prospect of a lifetime of suffering. But this apparently inescapable fate can often be averted by suitable therapy, and, in any case, it can be alleviated. Although it is now certain that the pre-disposition for an illness is an inherited fate, it is just as certain that the unfolding of the illness depends on circumstances of the environment. A "life in the realm of order," or a well-regulated life, as Bircher-Benner has formulated and taught it, is the most powerful help on the way to successful therapy—no "miracle cure," but a well-tested road to health.

The forces of life cannot grow in the system of the rheumatism-and-arthritis patient unless he first returns to a healthy way of life. Only then can the autonomous curative processes increase in intensity.

THE THERAPEUTIC DIET

At the beginning, the diet is limited for a number of weeks to uncooked fresh food only. This raw-food diet may be extended from 6-8 weeks for a seriously ill patient, and may last only 2-3 weeks in mild cases. It is very poor in animal proteins and fat. In cases of chronic arthritis these must actually be completely avoided for some period of time in most instances, as there usually is a tendency to allergy due to regulatory disorders, and careful avoidance of animal foods (dairy products, eggs, and meat) within the framework of a fresh-food diet has proved to be the most reliable way to obtain a reversal.

The fresh-food diet is kept absolutely free of stimulants such as coffee, alcohol, nicotine, and sweets so as not to weaken or neutralize its effect. This initiates the removal of sludge, reduction of synovial effusions, and loss of fluid in the soft connective tissues. These are then once again able to fulfill their important role of intermediary and selector in the process of assimilation and digestion and its regulatory function. The life processes of all tissues are strengthened by the rise in the cell potential. The potassium reserves increase. The centers of the nervous system recover, as do also the endocrine functions. But this will require time. It is important to overcome allergic tendencies. Typical of the rheumatic patient is the clotting of red blood cells which makes the blood flow sluggishly. It is assumed that this blood sludge stems from slackening body energy which is ideally restored through a raw-food diet. It is astonishing to observe how an organism begins to blossom out under the influence of this diet.

As soon as a satisfactory improvement is noted after 2-4 weeks of the strictly raw diet, whole-grain cooked cereals, vegetable bouillon, and potatoes boiled in their skins may be added. If improvement continues and settles at a certain level, the diet can be further expanded with the addition of various cooked vegetables, whole-grain bread and a little butter; after all allergic tendencies have disappeared mild white cheese, cottage cheese, yogurt, and sour milk may also be tried. The diet has to continue to remain low in sodium, low in fat, rich in fresh fruits and vegetables, and entirely free from the above-mentioned stimulants, of meat and processed foods. The patient is encouraged as he overcomes the crises of the first weeks and his condition gradually changes for the better; his confidence increases and he is pleased with the effective diet, and it is no longer necessary to keep urging him to persevere and be consistent.

Elimination of Seats of Infection

Chronic foci of infection—which mostly smolder away unnoticed—are apt to prevent the success of the treatment if they are not recognized and eliminated. It is therefore necessary to search for them in all rheumatic patients right at the start of the treatment. These foci can scatter toxins into the bloodstream which are then carried into the joints or other organs and cause or maintain inflammations. They continue to scatter bacterial poisons into the bloodstream which irritate the nervous system and hinder not only the overcoming of the allergic disposition, but also the recovery of the regulatory processes. The prime toxic foci in rheumatics are the tonsils (tonsilitis). The teeth also require careful attention and toxic foci there must be eliminated even if no direct connection between the focus and the inflammation of the joints can be demonstrated. The gall-bladder, too, can become an important focus of irritation and source of infection, even if its chronic inflammation takes its course without particularly distressing symptoms. The bowels can also serve as a source of infection if the normal coli flora has been supplanted by harmful bacteria and pus or if there is a chronic inflammation such as chronic appendicitis. A history of childhood diseases such as scrofula or tuberculosis should be examined further as they might have left behind an allergic and rheumatic stimulus although they might have been considered healed. Here, the fresh food diet can be very effective. It is often necessary to clear and disinfect the colon by colonic irrigation. If the healthy bacterial flora of the colon has been completely superseded, it is possible to assist recovery by introducing fresh coli cultures.

Physical Therapy

To the basic treatment through diet and the elimination of eventual foci of infection, physical treatment procedures are added in order to further the general and localized healing process. Their purpose is to promote the breathing of the skin, generally to improve the circulation, help a localized increase in the blood supply, and mobilize the patient's own defenses and restorative powers to the greatest possible extent.

Acute rheumatism is recognizable through the presence

of fever, reddening of the joint, pain accompanying the slightest movement, with pressure and at rest, swelling, and general discomfort including, sometimes, heart trouble. The goal of the treatment is, above all, a decrease in the inflammation and the temperature. This can be achieved through rest, compresses, cool water or clay packings, herbal and cabbage compresses (cabbage leaves are laid upon the skin under the wrappings), exposure to a mild sun lamp (no perspiring!), immobilization and correct positioning of the affected limbs on leafy or fern cushions. But a prerequisite is the above-mentioned therapeutic diet.

Rheumatism in its chronic stage is marked by absence of fever, coolness, and imperviousness to irritation, but stiffening, scarring, deformation, distortion of the muscles of the diseased parts of the body, and pain when the stiffened joints are moved. Treatment aims at promoting the flow of blood, loosening up tissues and joints, exercising the muscles, stimulating the circulation, increasing overall resistance, and overcoming allergic tendencies. This is achieved by means of hot herb, clay, sulfur, Aescusal, mud, or sometimes very hot baths, mud compresses, and most simply by light sweat-baths in bed, supplemented by massage of the joints and muscles and exercise therapy. Again the diet is the basis of the treatment. Because of its simplicity, the light-bath in bed is preferable to all other ways of heat application for rheumatism. Sweating as a cure has been used for ages. It causes a reduction in fluid retention, stimulates the body's defenses, and spurs the healing process. A light arc with eight electric bulbs is sufficient to send a continuous flow of warmth through the whole body or certain parts as needed (for climatic effect), or to induce sweating (10-15 minutes perspiration, then a brief dowsing of water, cold then steaming, and rest, wrapped in sheets). This simple treatment causes the arthritic's often rough and dry skin to become gradually soft again and supple, and the regenerative cycle of the skin is restored. It is usually possible to rent such light arcs from sick-bed supply houses, or they can be bought, which is economical because of their extended use.

Therapeutic baths

Baths to which vegetable or mineral therapeutic substances have been added, or natural therapeutic baths, which are available in a number of well known rheuma-spas, contribute most lastingly and intensively to the re-conditioning of the vegetative nervous system when they are combined with the diet described above. Such baths are: sulfur baths, mud baths, seaweed baths, Aescusal baths, Rheuhumin baths, radioactive baths, and many more. The effects of the Aescusal baths can be enhanced by rhythmic movement of the water, in the manner of a mild, but intensive tissue "massage." The organic and anorganic mineral additions to the baths, or their content in naturally therapeutic springs, are able to penetrate through the skin into the circulation and the diseased tissues and thus have a healthful effect. Under expert guidance, heated baths, sauna baths, alternate hot and cold baths, partial and half baths, clay compresses, clay and mud packings, can then be applied. Its application and dosage must be suited to the individual case, and should be supervised by an experienced physician. The numerous well-known hydrotherapeutic establishments, which can be found everywhere, as well as clubs, institutes, and books, are rich in appropriate expertise.

Hot-sand bath for the hands

If the finger joints are immobilized or deformed, a bowl of fine dry sand is heated and the patient "plays" in it with his hands. This is often very effective in improving mobility.

Massage

Massage should be used at the not acutely inflamed stage. This stimulates circulation, and in addition, the adhering layers of tissue are separated and can, again, move against each other. The condition of the tissues surrounding the joints is no less important for their mobility than that of the joint itself. It is also vitally important that the atrophied muscles be massaged. Special reflex-zone massage revives the circulation as well as the innervation of the affected limbs. All types of massage, in order to be properly effective, have to be carried out by professionally trained personnel. Acutely inflamed areas must not be massaged.

Gymnastics

Daily gymnastic exercise, which has been tailored to the patient's condition, gradually improves the functioning of the joints. It may require much perseverance before the patient can release himself from his wheelchair, and then from his canes, and before he can finally walk upright; but when all the above measures interact, this goal is reached most rapidly. The patient needs consistent and experienced guidance and loving encouragement to give him the patience, persistence, and courage to persevere.

Electrical treatments

Diathermy (Novodyn, Iontophoresis): These treatments are applied where deep local heat penetration and stimulation are desired. *X-ray radiation:* Radiation should be used cautiously (because of its side effects); it may be applied as a last resort in certain otherwise unresponsive changes in the joints, often with good results, when everything else has failed.

MEDICATION

The multiplicity of causes which act together in rheumatic disease suggest caution, particularly in combining medications. Many remedies, which at first seem to promise certain success, yet do not provide the desired *permanent* improvement. An improvement in their therapeutic action is often noted when the unspecific natural therapeutic methods are applied simultaneously, owing to elimination of their side effects. Without medical prescription and control, the patient should not take any medication under any circumstance. Medication is always only a bridge, an emergency measure, to be used for the shortest possible time, and never the basis of the treatment. This is not the place to enter into details on the uses of specific medications; the choice of a medication is up to the physician.

Homeopathic treatment carried out with medical expertise, can also be a very valuable and effective addition to the basic treatment.

Localized treatment of rheumatism with rheumatism ointments, Spanish fly plaster, leeches and similar bloodletting devices can increase the flow of blood and improve immunologic responses, but here also—not without a doctor!

Neurotherapy: Treatment with Impletol according to the German Dr. Kuneke can, under expert handling, promote the healing process neurologically by eliminating the localized pain perception through a careful injection of Novocain into the exact nerve points where the pain is felt, as in acupuncture and nerve massage.

Active immunization may be induced by the method developed by Dr. von Ponndorf, with the injection of Rheumacutin B. This mobilizes the dormant resistance of the organism. In conjunction with the basic treatment, it can lead to spectacular results.

Acupuncture and *electro-puncture* are very interesting and valuable, and bring good results. However, they require many years of specialized training and experience and should only be done by experts.

Prophylaxis and Prevention of Relapses

Varied as the causes may be which contribute to the inception of rheumatic diseases, in the last instance they are all based on departures from a naturally ordered way of life. For this reason, Dr. Bircher-Benner wrote, shortly before his death, when he was devoting his last strength to the problem of rheumatic disease: *"There is a safe and reliable way to prevent rheumatic diseases: a naturally ordered way of life."*

Today, when the excesses of frantic work, excitement, impressions, food and drink, stimulations, and amusements, undermine the resistance against disease with which man has been amply provided; when our diet is generally far too poor in vital substances and valuable fresh raw foods and much too rich in animal fats, protein, sugar, refined flour, and added preservatives, and adulterated to boot; where man, all too often, cannot get around to profound experiences, to a realization of essential values and truth, and to genuine, creative activity; where lack of exercise, fresh air, and sufficient sleep further undermine his vitality—he often finds himself trapped in a truly vicious circle, from which no "elixir" or "wonder drug" will release him, but only the return to a wholesome way of life. This is the simple truth, and it is the natural path which the aware, and only he himself, can take. This has to be understood by anyone who has recovered from serious rheumatic disease and who wants to avoid a relapse into renewed illness. This must also be understood by those who wish to protect them, and their own, from the sad fate of similar illness.

The rule of order begins first with the *rhythm of the day:* "early to rise and early to bed." The increase in vitality and productivity this brings about is astonishing. The autonomous nervous system, in its alternation between "high gear" and "low gear," is adjusted to the rhythm of the natural world (day and night), and is used up much too fast if night is turned into day and vice versa. An adequate lunch break is recommended: a leisurely meal, plus a minimum of ½ hour's rest preferably lying down.

Adequate physical exercise

Some of the dominant requirements at the present time are walking to work instead of driving, or *walking* in the morning, before the air is polluted by exhaust fumes. More extensive walks (2-3 hours) in the woods and mountains on weekends are desirable.

Take all opportunities to *breathe* deeply *by the open window,* stretch and bend all joints, in light gymnastics and sports (swimming, rowing). A daily air bath is required

(5 minutes) at all times of the year, where the skin over the entire body is massaged gently with dry brushes until it glows. If possible *sun baths* (the skin needs sun): begin systematically with 5 minutes on each side, gradually increase to 20 minutes on each side. Protect the head from sun. Always top off with a cold shower. Such sensible sun baths have an astringent effect on the skin: it becomes velvety soft, and the entire organism is rejuvenated. *Hot and cold showers* strengthen the body and give a sense of well-being: daily 1-2-3 minutes hot and then 20-40 seconds cold, alternate 2-3 times. Result: intensive reddening of the skin, tiredness disappears. Baths should not be too long or too hot. A rheumatism-prone person generally recoils from cold. However he more than any other is in need of intensive reactivation of his weakened responses to cold stimulation. He must not dress too warmly. He has to proceed carefully, and step by step, and must take care that he is always comfortably warmed through before and after the conditioning cold stimulus. *Cold showers* with forceful sprays over arms and legs are wonderfully refreshing but should never be used after coming straight out of bed or without preceding warming-up and exercise. Sleeplessness may be fought by nightly "foot baths" in a bucket of cold water. Headaches and congestion of the blood vessels in the head can be helped with *warm-and-cold foot baths:* take 2 deep buckets, one filled with water at 102 degrees F (calf deep, add hot water as needed), the other with tap water. Soak feet for 5-10 minutes in hot water, then for 10-20-40 seconds in cold water, alternate about three times, finish with cold water. Selectron baths have a similar effect.

Permanent diet

Particularly serious offenses against the natural order of living are today committed in the field of daily nutrition. For prophylaxis and prevention of a relapse in patients with a rheumatic disposition, a diet is recommended which, though by no means as restricted as the above-mentioned therapeutic diet, should yet be very rich in fresh natural foods (fresh raw fruit, raw vegetables, nuts, perhaps full milk, together at least half of the daily food intake). For the rest, whole-grain foods, vegetables, and potatoes (lightly cooked) and dairy products. On the whole the meals should be sparing, normally not more than one main meal and 2 light meals. Care and attention should be devoted to flavor and taste. Stimulants, desserts, sweets, foods overly rich in fat and protein (meat!) only on *exceptional* occasions, never as a daily habit! The desire for it soon disappears, so the sacrifice is no genuine sacrifice any more. The pleasure found in self-control and in the newly discovered tastes and flavors, above all the enjoyment of a steady pleasantly-fresh vitality which had been all but forgotten, are ample compensations. The weight should be controlled and a watch kept on the patient's general condition: whenever the weight increases or decreases significantly beyond normal limits, the diet is reintroduced for a short period.

All this, however, will hardly succeed and suffice unless one central feature is added: it is necessary to regain a clear view of the hour, the day, and life as a whole, and learn to stand above the things, and cease being an over-conscientious and compulsively dutiful harried slave, to become instead the serene ruler and master of one's life. To achieve this, it is necessary to *consider the essentials* at the beginning and at the end of each day and to have a daily schedule which allows time for contemplation and creative self-development, and for a satisfying and rich relationship with the inner and outer world. If overstimulation of the vegetative nervous system has become too extensive and persistent, it is recommended to study, with a good teacher, contemplative self-realization in the form of autogenous training or Yoga. The crux of such practice is the alternation of deep conscious inhalation, and exhalation with the diaphragm completely relaxed, which is wonderfully soothing. After some practice, many problems decrease in importance and one makes constant progress in learning to stand above common matters. Periods of rest have to be scheduled in every phase of a busy and active life. This is more than ever essential where life is full of agitation, tension, and constant excitement and soul and emotions get short shrift.

IV. Recipes

The physician's instructions must depend on the degree of the illness, as to how constrictive a diet should be followed. The pure raw-food diet should be followed by rheumatics for at least 2-8 weeks. For the transitional and permanent diet, see Bircher-Benner's cookbook *Eating Your Way to Health* published by Penguin Books, in an American edition; Baltimore, Maryland: 1972.

For the strict diet, only the recipes not marked by an asterisk (*) should be considered; all the recipes may be used in milder diets.

Muesli

1. The Apple Muesli*

The original Apple Muesli first introduced by Dr. Bircher Benner has, in our long experience, remained the outstanding and best dietary food.

In general, it is best to use the tart, white fleshed, juicy variety of apples such as Gravenstein, Jonathan, McIntosh, Winesaps, Rhode Island Greening, Cortland, Red and Golden Delicious.

If the season is advanced, and drier or less tasty varieties have to be used, their flavor can be enriched by the addition of freshly grated orange or lemon peel, if unsprayed is available, by adding orange juice immediately before serving and, also, occasionally, by the addition of a little rose-hip puree.

1 level tbsp. rolled oats
3 tbsp. cold water
1 tbsp. lemon juice
1 tbsp. condensed milk, unsweetened
1-2 tbsp. water as needed, depending on type of apples
1/2 lb. apples
1 tsp. honey or fruit concentrate
1 tbsp. ground hazelnuts or almonds

Soak oats for 12 hours in water. (Do not soak instant oats, but use same amount of water.) Add juice, milk, water and combine into smooth sauce. Wash apples, dry with clean cloth, remove stem and blossom end. Grate apples (on Bircher grater—obtainable at health-food stores) straight into the sauce, stirring frequently to avoid discoloration of pulp. Grate apples as soon as possible before serving. Sprinkle nuts over sauce before serving.

The following may be substituted for one tbsp. rolled oats:

   1 tsp. rolled oats, soaked, 1 tsp. corn kernels (soak in water for 24 hours, then pour into sieve, rinse with cold water). The kernels may be whole, shredded, or mixed.
   Wheat, rice, barley, rye, millet, buckwheat, or soy flakes may also be used; also the ground, dried wheatflakes available in health stores; yeast flakes may be added for vitamin-B enrichment.

2. Apple Muesli with Almond Puree or Sesame Puree

1 level tbsp. rolled oats
3 tbsp. water
1 tbsp. lemon juice
1 tbsp. almond puree or sesame puree
1 tbsp. honey or raw sugar
3 tbsp. water
1/2 lb. apples
1 tbsp. ground hazelnuts or almonds

Soak oats for 12 hours in water. Combine and thoroughly mix remaining ingredients with wire whisk, except apples and nuts. Prepare apples as in basic recipe No. 1. Sprinkle nuts over dish before serving.

3. Apple Muesli with Yogurt*

1 level tbsp. rolled oats
3 tbsp. water
3 tbsp. yogurt
1 tsp. lemon juice
1 tbsp. honey
1/2 lb. apples
1 tbsp. ground hazelnuts or almonds

Soak oats for 12 hours in water. Combine with yogurt, lemon juice, honey and beat into a smooth sauce. Prepare apples as in basic recipe No. 1. Sprinkle nuts over dish before serving.

4. Muesli with Berries or Pitted Fruit

Especially rich in vitamin C; wash fruit thoroughly.

5-8 oz. well-ripened strawberries
or raspberries, blueberries, red currants, blackberries
or 5-8 oz. plums, peaches, apricots
(Prepare sauce as in recipe No. 2.)

Mash berries with wooden pestle or fork, or grind pitted fruit in chromed mincer or mince finely with knife.

5. Muesli with Various Fruit Combinations

Strawberries and raspberries
Strawberries, raspberries, and currants
Strawberries and apples
Blackberries and apples
Apples with finely chopped orange and tangerine slivers
Apples and bananas
Plums and peaches or apricots, etc.
(Prepare sauce as in recipe No. 2.)

(Apricots and plums should be avoided when stomach or intestinal disease is present.)

6. Muesli with Dried Fruit

If circumstances demand that Muesli be prepared with dried fruit (apples, apricots, prunes), wash 4 oz. dried fruit per portion, soak in cold water for 12 hrs., and run through grinder. Combine this mixture with the sauce given in the basic recipe.

When using dried fruit, it is important to insist on good quality, without bleach and preservatives to prevent undesirable stomach and bowel upsets.

Raw Vegetables

Four basic rules must be observed in preparing raw vegetables:

1. Freshness: It is best to use sun-ripened, organically grown vegetables; if possible they should be home grown.

Raw vegetables should be prepared as soon as possible before consumption, to avoid wilting and loss of juices, and so that contact of the shredded vegetables with air should be as short as possible. (Mix quickly into the sauce)

2. Quality: By quality it is understood that leafy and root vegetables should be young and tender, not bleached but fully ripe in coloring; the fertilizer used should be balanced and not excessive, with compost if possible; and the plants should be free of disease. This is particularly important in a diet for sick people.

3. Thorough Cleaning: In order to prevent worms and infection by colibacilli, the following instructions for cleaning vegetables should be strictly followed.

Vegetables grown organically and without liquid manure do not contain worm eggs.

4. Well-balanced Combinations: Each meal of raw vegetables should, if possible, consist of root, fruit, and leafy vegetables. A therapeutic diet, in particular, should not lack green-leafed vegetables. The sameness of the all-raw-vegetable dish should also be relieved by a variety of dressings.

A three-color scheme enhances the appearance of the salad and adds to the enjoyment of eating.

Small decorations made of herbs, radishes, young carrots, etc. may be used on special occasions to give the raw-vegetable dish a more colorful and festive look, but in general there should not be more than three different raw vegetables per meal; it is preferable to provide variety during the course of the day. Too much diversity can have a bad effect on digestion.

The Cleaning of Leafy Vegetables

Iceberg lettuce, endives, Boston or leaf lettuce, savoy cabbage, cabbage, red cabbage, escarole, etc. Separate the leaves, remove brown and damaged parts and soak in salt water (1 handful of salt to 1-1/2 gallons of water) for 1 hour. Rinse repeatedly; if possible wash each leaf separately under a jet of water. Dry in a wire basket or with a clean dry cloth.

Escarole, spinach, dandelion, watercress, Brussels sprouts and similar small-leafed vegetables require special care in preparation and cleaning. Rinse repeatedly in small amounts, remove small roots and tough stems. Cut chicory and endive in half, remove outer leaves and rinse thoroughly.

The Cleaning of Root Vegetables

Celery roots, carrots, viper's grass, beets, black radish, kohlrabi, white and red radishes. The roots should be cleaned with a vegetable brush under running water. Peel and place immediately in cold water to which salt and lemon juice have been added (1/2 lemon to 1-1/2 gallons of water) to preserve the fresh color of the vegetables.

The Cleaning of Vegetable Fruits

Tomatoes, cucumbers, zucchini, bell peppers. The washed fruit may be peeled or cut into slices and small pieces.

Cucumbers should be peeled from the center out; cut off bitter ends. Tender cucumbers may be eaten unpeeled.

For salads, only young and tender zucchini should be used; unpeeled. Green and yellow peppers are less sharp than the red ones. Halve the peppers and remove the seeds; slice the thick parts and soak in water if they are too sharp.

Cut the cauliflower flowerets into fairly large pieces, remove damaged parts, peel the stems lightly and soak in salt water. Scrape celery stalks, remove tough parts. Halve leeks, prepare, and wash under running water. Halve fennel and wash.

Special Cleaning Methods

If doubts exist concerning the cleanliness and freedom from contamination of vegetables or fruits (especially in southern and tropical countries), the following cleansing methods are to be followed:

1. To free the vegetables from worm eggs and insects, soak them in a weak salt solution (1 handful of cooking salt to 5 quarts of water). The salt solution dissolves the protein layer by which the worm eggs are attached, and rinsing later removes them.

2. Bacteria, colibacilli, and fungi, which are not dangerous to healthy people in our geographical regions, may be removed with *citric acid* or vinegar. Dissolve 2 oz. of citric acid (obtainable in drug stores) in 1 quart of water and soak the vegetables, especially the leafy ones, for 15 minutes in this solution. Then rinse thoroughly under running water. Pour off citric acid solution and store: it can be used again 3 to 4 times.

3. Root and fruit vegetables are prepared and put into a sieve which is immersed in boiling water for 10 seconds. This makes the surface germ free, and yet leaves the inside of the vegetable raw.

4. Vegetable and fruit juices are rendered practically germ free, even without these preparations, by the addition of 1/5 of the juice of a *freshly squeezed* lemon.

5. For protection from amoebic infection in the tropics,

the prepared vegetables are dipped into a solution of chloride of lime (1 tsp. chloride of lime to 1 quart of water). Remove chloride of lime by rinsing with boiled water.

Salad Dressings

7. Oil Dressing

1 tbsp. oil
1 tsp. lemon juice
Onion or garlic
1 tsp. fresh or dried herbs

Mix everything together well.

8. Mayonnaise Dressing

Makes 6-8 servings of mayonnaise.

1 egg yolk, whisked
1 cup of oil
A few drops of lemon juice

Add oil to egg yolk drop by drop, beating constantly with egg whisk. Add lemon juice to thin.

For 1 serving of mayonnaise dressing:

1 tbsp. mayonnaise
1 tsp. lemon juice
A little onion or garlic
1 tsp. fresh or
1 pinch dried herbs

Mix all ingredients together well.

9. Mayonnaise Dressing/with Soy Flour Instead of Egg

2 level tbsp. soy flour
6 tbsp. water

3/4 cup oil
3 tbsp. lemon juice

Mix soy flour and water into smooth dough. Alternately, add oil and lemon juice slowly while constantly beating with egg whisk.

For 1 serving:

Same procedure as for mayonnaise sauce.

10. Cream Dressing*

2 tbsp. cream
1 tsp. cottage cheese
1 tsp. lemon juice
A little onion or garlic
1 tsp. fresh or
1 pinch dried herbs

Mix all ingredients together thoroughly with egg whisk.

11. Yogurt Dressing*

2-3 tbsp. yogurt
Some drops of lemon juice
A little onion or garlic
1 tsp. fresh or
1 pinch dried herbs

Mix all ingredients together thoroughly with egg whisk.

12. Almond or Sesame Puree Dressing*

1 tbsp. almond puree or sesame puree
3 tbsp. water
1 tsp. lemon juice
A little onion or garlic
1 tsp. fresh or
1 pinch dried herbs

Stir puree slowly with water; add remaining ingredients.

The Following Salads and Raw Vegetables†

13. Boston lettuce	Do not cut into small pieces
14. Cos lettuce	Do not cut into small pieces
15. Endives	Cut into 1/3" strips
16. Romaine lettuce	Cut into 1/3" strips
17. Dandelion greens	Do not cut up
18. Watercress	Do not cut up
19. Spinach	Cut into 1/6" strips
20. Head salads: White cabbage, sauerkraut, Brussel sprouts, savoy and Chinese cabbage	shred, cut into fine strips
21. Tomatoes	Slice or dice
22. Cucumbers	Grate
23. Fennel	Cut fine with knife and shred
24. Peppers	Cut in fine strips
25. White radish	Grate or shred
26. Radishes	Grate
27. Celery sticks	Cut fine
28. Zucchini	Grate into fine slices or shred coarsely
29. Carrots	Shred fine
30. Celery root	Shred fine
31. Beets	Shred fine or coarse
32. Cauliflower	Cut off flowers, shred stems
33. Chicory	Cut into 1/3" strips
34. Jerusalem Artichoke	Shred
35. Kohlrabi	Shred fine or grate
36. Red cabbage	Grate or shred fine

---

† For cleaning of vegetables, see Raw Vegetables, pages 32-35.

Are Prepared With:

oil dressing		chives, onions
oil dressing		chives, onions
oil dressing	or mayonnaise*	chives, onions, parsley†
oil dressing	or mayonnaise*	basil, marjoram*
oil dressing	or mayonnaise*	onion
oil dressing	or mayonnaise*	onion
oil dressing	or mayonnaise*	mint
oil dressing	or mayonnaise*	rosemary, savory, thyme, caraway seeds
oil dressing	or mayonnaise*	basil, thyme, dill
oil dressing	or mayonnaise*	dill
oil dressing	or mayonnaise*	onion, chives
oil dressing	or mayonnaise*	chives
oil dressing		chives
oil dressing		chives
oil dressing		onion, chives
oil dressing	or mayonnaise*	dill, borage, basil
almond puree	or oil dressing	marjoram, rosemary
almond puree	or oil dressing	basil, thyme
almond puree	or mayonnaise	rosemary, thyme, caraway
almond puree	or mayonnaise	basil, marjoram, nutmeg
almond puree	or oil dressing	tarragon, marjoram
almond puree		thyme, spearmint
almond puree	or oil dressing	thyme, rosemary
almond puree	or oil dressing	grated apple, caraway, rosemary

---

† Chives, parsley, and onions may be added to all raw vegetables in moderation.

37. Raw Vegetables, Mixed

Chicory with diced tomatoes—oil dressing or mayon-
naise*
Peppers and fennel—oil dressing
Fennel, chicory and diced tomatoes—almond purée
dressing or mayonnaise
Fennel and carrots—almond purée dressing
Cauliflower and carrots—almond purée dressing
Tomatoes and peppers—oil dressing or almond purée
dressing

38. Tomatoes, Raw, Stuffed

With cucumbers—oil dressing or mayonnaise*
With celery—almond puree dressing
With cauliflower—almond puree dressing
With white cabbage—mayonnaise

39. Grains, Sprouted

*Especially high vitamins E and B content group. Very
nutritious.*

Wheat, rye, oats, barley.
1st day, evening: Wash grains in sieve under running
water and place in small dish. Cover with water at room
temperature, near heater.
2nd day, morning: Rinse and dry on a flat plate at room
temperature near heater. Evening: Replace in a small dish
again and cover with water at room temperature, near
heater.
3rd day, morning: Rinse, dry, and spread on a plate. Evening: Put in a small dish and cover with water at room
temperature, near heater.
By this time, the grains should have germinated and developed shoots 1/3 to 2/3 of an inch in length.

40. Especially for Children

Shredded grain is soaked, mixed with bananas, honey, and water.

Sauerkraut

This raw vegetable is particularly valuable, especially in winter. It is more easily digested raw than cooked**. If steamed sauerkraut is served, its flavor and digestibility can be improved by the addition of a little shredded fresh sauerkraut.

Sauerkraut Salad

The sauerkraut is loosened up and cut small, and mixed with caraway seeds (or also ground caraway), 3-4 small chopped juniper berries, chopped onion, and an apple which has been cut into small strips. Sprinkle with the juice of 1 lemon and 2 tbsp. olive oil. Serve with lettuce and any kind of raw vegetables.

Juices

High-grade bottled berry, fruit, and vegetable juice may be obtained in health-food stores, if it is too difficult to prepare them at home.

Raw nutrients mechanically refined, such as juices, are added as special enrichment and where roughage (cellulose) is forbidden as in stomach and intestinal disease. It should, however, be borne in mind that the original raw food is always more valuable and cannot be permanently replaced by juices. For this reason, the patient should return to fruit and raw vegetables as soon as possible.

General: Cleaning, see introduction in chapter on raw vegetables. A variety of juicers are sold, from the small manual juicer to the motorized centrifuge for the prepa-

---

** Ask for low-sodium sauerkraut at your health-food store.

ration of fruit and vegetable juices. If a manual juicer is used, it is first necessary to cut the fruits and vegetables into small pieces. Apples, pears, and all root vegetables must be finely grated; leafy vegetables and herbs must be chopped into very small pieces.

41. Fruit Juices

Fruits for juice are served immediately after squeezing. Every delay means a loss in food value.

a) *Unmixed Fruit Juices* (nothing added):

Oranges, tangerines, grapefruit, apples, pears, grapes, strawberries, blueberries, currants, raspberries, peaches, apricots, plums.

b) *Mixed Fruit Juices:*

Oranges, tangerines, grapefruit, persimmon, or
Berry juice with apple juice or
Berry juice with peach, apricot, or plum juice
Bananas, whipped, with orange, berry, peach, apricot juice.

Additions, according to taste or instructions: Lemon juice, raw sugar, honey, fruit concentrate, cream*, yogurt, almond milk, linseed, rice, or barley purée.

42. Vegetable Juices

Serve these juices fresh for their high mineral and vitamin content. Each juice has a specific value of its own.

a) *Unmixed Vegetable Juices:*

Tomatoes, carrots, beets, white radish, cabbage, celery, potatoes, all leafy, tuberous, and root vegetables.

b) *Mixed Vegetable Juices:*

In our experience, the best combinations are:

> Carrots, tomatoes, spinach (in equal parts)
> Tomato and carrot
> Tomato and spinach
> Other combinations (and cocktails) may be prepared according to individual taste.

For variety, add juices of the following: sorrel, nettle, chives, parsley, onion, tender celery leaves or roots, and other herbs.

Add per glass (1/2-2/3 fluid oz.): 1 tsp. almond puree, some lemon juice, perhaps a little fruit concentrate, or linseed, rice, or barley puree. Other leafy vegetables or salad greens may also be used, e.g., white cabbage, Savoy cabbage, lettuce, endives, collard, Romaine lettuce, dandelion. In spring, the blood can be cleansed by the addition of nettle, sorrel, and dandelion juice.

c) *Potato Juice:*

> Use only thoroughly cleaned potatoes, peeled or unpeeled (do not use greenish, unripe, or sprouted potatoes).

Prepare like carrot juice. It may have a rather unpleasant taste. Take it on doctor's orders.

43. Purees as Additions to Juices

To be added to other raw juices (1 part of puree to 2 parts juice); it neutralizes the acid fruit taste.

a) *Rice or Barley Gruel:*

> 1 heaped tsp. rice or barley flour
> 4/5 cup of water

Combine ingredients cold, and boil for 5 minutes, stirring constantly. Let cool.

b)   *Linseed Gruel:*

    1 tbsp. linseed
    4/5 cup of water

Wash, and boil linseed in water for 10 minutes. Strain off and let cool.

One day's supply may be prepared once daily and stored in a thermos bottle, to be added to all raw juices.

Varieties of Non-Dairy Milk

44. Almond Milk

A vegetable protein-fat food, mucilaginous and soothing.

    1 tbsp. almond puree
    2 tsp. honey
    5 oz. water
    5 oz. water and 1-1/2 oz. fruit juice produces slightly
       thicker mixture

Stir almond puree and honey together with an egg whisk and add water drop by drop.

45. Almond Milk Made from Fresh Almonds

Very easy to digest.

    1-1/2 tbsp. almonds, peeled
    1 tsp. honey
    5 oz. water

Mix in mixer or blender. Strained. (No bitter almonds!)

46. Pine Nut Milk

Very rich in easily digested fat and vegetable protein.

1-1/2 tbsp. pine nuts, washed
1 tsp. honey
5 oz. water

Prepare as almond milk.

47. Sesame Milk

7 oz. water (cold or warm—according to taste)
1 level tbsp. sesame puree
1 tsp. lemon juice.
1 tsp. raw sugar or honey

Beat sesame puree and sugar or honey together with an egg whisk, and add water drop by drop.

48. Cream of Sesame

Prepare as sesame milk, but with less water. For cold dishes or as a cream substitute.

49. Sesame Frappe

Prepare as sesame milk or cream of sesame, with the addition of fruit juice, sweet cider, fruit concentrates, etc.

50. Bircher Muesli with Sesame Puree

See Bircher Muesli, recipe No. 2.

51. Mayonnaise with Sesame Puree

See salad dressings.

52. Soy Milk

Wash and dry soy beans, grind like almonds.

    1/2 cup soy beans
    3-1/2 cups water
    1 tbsp. sugar
    water

Soak for 2 hours; then boil for 20 minutes in the same water, stirring steadily. Strain, add water until mixture reaches cow's milk consistency. Add sugar, and let cool.

Butter, Vegetable Fats, and Oils

53. We use

Fresh Butter: Used to refine the food and most recipes in the diets.

Nussella†: A mixture of coconut fat, sunflower oil, and olive oil, rather like melted butter.

Vegetable Margarine and Fats: Vegetable-fat emulsions from natural hard fats such as coconut oil or palm-kernel oil together with the largest possible proportion of liquid oils and seed oils—especially sunflower-seed oil.

Nut and almond purees: Has the finest nutty flavor and has many uses in bland diets; also, in place of fresh butter with vegetables, potatoes, rice, noodles, etc.

Cold-Pressed Sunflower Oil, Corn-germ Oil, Linseed Oil, Olive Oil: Carefully processed, rich in poly-unsaturated fatty acids; these are very valuable fats

---

† Nussella is a Swiss brand name.

owing to their purity, and are generally more easily digested than melted butter.

Soups

The Recipes Given Are for One Serving

We use a great deal of vegetable stock in our soup and vegetable recipes. In a small household, where it is not possible to prepare fresh stock every day, ordinary water may be substituted, and liquid health-store yeast germ or vegetarian salt-free vegetable-bouillon cubes may be used to add flavor. Cream improves any soup and any vegetable; however, milk can be used in place of cream in most instances.

Health-food-store yeast extracts are yeast products very rich in vitamin B (rich in glutathione and lecithin).

54. Vegetable Stock

This is the only recipe calculated for 4 servings. Select the vegetables according to the season, e.g., celery, carrots, some cabbage or kohlrabi, leek, tomatoes, and onions. Tough, but healthy vegetable parts, such as potato skins etc., may also be used.

1 tbsp. vegetable fat
1 onion
2 carrots
1 small celery root (5 oz.)
Collards, Swiss chard, cabbage
1 leek
3-4 quarts cold water
Rosemary, basil, or other fresh or dried herbs
1/2 bay leaf
1 pinch salt

Melt fat. Halve onions without removing skin and brown cut surfaces thoroughly. Cut vegetables into small pieces and add to onions. Cover and simmer for at least 1/4 hour over small flame. Add water and simmer for 2 hours on small flame. Season to taste.

55. Vegetable Bouillon

10 oz. vegetable stock
A little brewer's yeast extract if desired
2 tsp. nut puree
Season with: Parsley, chives, finely chopped herbs.

Pour hot vegetable stock over nut puree and herbs.

56. Sago Soup with Vegetables

1 tbsp. sago
1 pint vegetable stock
1/2 tbsp. vegetable fat
1 small diced carrot
1 small celery root, diced
1 small leek, cut in strips
1 pinch salt
Season with: Brewer's yeast extract, parsley, chives.

Stir sago into boiling vegetable stock. Sauté vegetables in fat until tender, add to vegetable stock and simmer for 1/2 hour. Add salt.

57. Rice Soup, Clear

1/2 tbsp. vegetable fat
2 cups vegetable stock
1 small onion, chopped
1 small carrot, thinly sliced
Celery root, thinly sliced
Leek, thinly sliced
1 tbsp. rice
1 pinch salt

Melt fat. Sauté onion in fat. Add vegetables and rice to stock and simmer all together. Add salt.

58. Rice Soup, Thick

1/2 tbsp. vegetable fat
Celery root, finely cut
Small carrot, sliced thin
1 leek, sliced
1 tbsp. rice
1/2 tbsp. flour
2-1/4 cups vegetable stock or water
1/2 tbsp. cream
1 pinch salt
Chives
Season with: Brewer's yeast extract, rosemary, parsley,
    basil, marjoram

Sauté vegetables in melted fat. Sprinkle flour on vegetable mixture. Add stock and simmer for 30 minutes. Put cream into soup bowl, and add soup. Add salt. Sprinkle chives over individual bowl.

59. Cream of Rice

1 tbsp. rice flour
1/4 tbsp. flour
3 tbsp. milk*
2-1/4 cups vegetable stock
1/2 tbsp. butter or nut puree
1 tbsp. cream*
1 pinch salt
Season with: Chives, marjoram, nutmeg or caraway.

Stir together flour and milk and add to boiling vegetable stock. Simmer 1/2 hr. Put butter into soup bowl and pour soup over it. Add salt and cream.

60. Herb Soup

1 tbsp. flour
6 tbsp. milk*
2 cups vegetable stock
1 tbsp. cream*
1 tsp. butter or nut puree if desired
1 pinch salt
Season with: Rosemary, basil, tarragon, marjoram,
    chives; also, nutmeg or caraway.

Mix flour with a little cold milk and stir into boiling vegetable stock; simmer 1/4 hr. Stir cream and butter into boiling soup. Add salt.

61. Soy Soup

1 tbsp. vegetable fat
A little onion
1 tbsp. flour
1/2 tbsp. soy flour
1/2 peeled, diced tomato
2 cups vegetable stock
1 pinch salt.
Season with: Basil, marjoram, or rosemary, chives,
    parsley.

Sauté onion in melted vegetable fat. Add flour and soy flour. Add tomato, stock, and salt last.

62. Cream of Oats Soup

1/2 tbsp. vegetable fat
1/2 tbsp. flour
2 tbsp. rolled oats
2-1/4 cups vegetable stock
1 piece celery or celeriac

1 pinch salt
1 tbsp. cream
Season with: Brewer's yeast extract, chives, nutmeg
 or caraway if desired.

Brown flour and oats slightly in melted fat. Add stock, celery, and salt. Simmer 1 hour. Strain. Put cream into soup bowl and pour soup over it.

63. Groats Soup

1/2 tbsp. vegetable fat
Chopped onion
2 tbsp. groats
3 cups water or vegetable stock
2/3 cup milk
Piece of celery
1 pinch salt
Brewer's yeast extract
1 tbsp. cream* if desired
Season with: Chives, parsley, marjoram or borage.

Sauté onion until yellow. Add groats and sauté until golden brown. Add stock, milk, celery and salt. Cook for 1 hour. Put yeast and cream into soup bowl, and pour soup over them.

64. Green Rye (Spelt) Soup

1/2 tbsp. vegetable fat
Chopped onion
1 tbsp. leek, chopped fine
Celery root, diced fine
1-2 tbsp. spelt (whole or shredded), soaked for 12 hrs.
6 tbsp. water
2 cups vegetable stock
1 pinch of salt
Season with: Rosemary (or finely chopped, fresh celery greens).

Sauté onion, leek, celery root. Cook thoroughly. Add spelt and sauté for a short time. Add water, salt, and stock and cook for 1-1/2 hours. Soup may be strained.

65. Swiss Semolina (Farina) Soup

1/2 tbsp. vegetable fat
1 tbsp. semolina (Farina)
1/2 tbsp. wholewheat flour
2 tbsp. Savoy cabbage, thinly sliced
2-1/2 cups vegetable stock
1 pinch salt
1 tbsp. cream*
1 tsp. fresh butter or nut puree
Season with: Brewer's yeast extract, finely chopped caraway, 1 clove nutmeg, if desired, rosemary, basil, marjoram, parsley, chives.

Sauté lightly semolina (farina) and whole wheat flour. Add cabbage and sauté until it is limp. Add stock and salt, and simmer for 1/2 hour. Put cream and butter into soup bowl and pour soup over them.

66. Brown Wholewheat Soup

1/2 tbsp. vegetable fat
1 tbsp. wholewheat flour
1 tbsp. flour
2-1/2 cups vegetable stock, cold
1/4 onion
Caraway seeds
1 pinch of salt
2 tsp. butter or nut puree
1 tbsp. cream* if desired
1 tbsp. grated cheese*
Season with: Small bay leaf, perhaps nutmeg, clove, marjoram, brewer's yeast.

Brown flour until nut brown and let cool. Stir in cold stock until smooth. Add onion, caraway seeds, and salt, and simmer 1/2 hour. Put butter, cream, and cheese into soup tureen, and pour soup over all.

67. Tomato Soup I

1/2 tbsp. vegetable fat
Onion (small amount)
Small carrot
1 stalk celery
1/2 leek
1 clove garlic
Rosemary
1 tomato
1 tbsp. flour
2-1/2 cups vegetable stock
1 pinch salt
Tomato puree to taste
1 tsp. butter or nut puree
1 tbsp. cream*
Season with: Sugar, clove, chives, bay leaf.
1 tbsp. rice, sago, or roasted croutons may be added.

Melt fat. Cut up all vegetables, except tomatoes, and sauté thoroughly. Add tomato. Sprinkle flour and sauté together. Add stock, cook 1/2 hour. Strain. Put butter and cream into a soup bowl and pour soup over all.

68. Tomato Soup II

4 ripe tomatoes
1 tsp. lemon juice
1 pinch of salt
1 tsp. sugar, if desired
1-1/2 tbsp. cream*

Cut tomatoes into pieces, add sugar and salt. Bring to a boil and strain. Add lemon juice or cream and serve soup lukewarm or cold.

69. Carrot Soup

1/2 tbsp. vegetable fat
1/2 onion, chopped
1 carrot, sliced
1-1/2 tbsp. flour
1 pinch salt
2 cups vegetable stock
6 tbsp. milk*
1 tsp. caraway seeds
Celery leaves or rosemary
1 tbsp. cream*
Season with: Rosemary or marjoram.

Melt fat. Sauté onion and carrot. Sprinkle flour over mixture and sauté together lightly. Add stock, milk, salt, caraway seeds, and celery. Simmer 1/2 hour and strain. Put cream in soup bowl and pour soup over it.

70. Spinach Soup

1/2 tbsp. vegetable fat
A little onion
1/2 clove garlic
1-1/2 tbsp. flour
2 cups vegetable stock
6 tbsp. milk*
1 cup spinach
Several mint leaves
1 pinch of salt
1 tbsp. cream*
Nutmeg
Season with: Parsley, chives, brewer's yeast
    extract, or sage leaves.

Sauté onion, garlic, and flour in melted fat. Add stock, milk, and salt and boil for 20 minutes. Chop spinach and mint leaves and add to finished soup (do not boil). Put cream and nutmeg into soup bowl and pour soup over both.

71. Califlower Soup

Several cauliflower clusters
1/2 tbsp. vegetable fat
1-1/2 tbsp. flour
2 cups vegetable stock
1 pinch of salt
Point of bay leaf
A little basil
1 tbsp. cream*
Season with: Brewer's yeast extract, parsley,
    chives, tarragon or nutmeg.

Cook cauliflower floret clusters separately. Cut stems (uncooked) into small pieces. Melt fat and sauté flour. Add stems and sauté together. Add stock, salt, bay leaf, and basil and simmer for 3/4 hour. Strain. Place cauliflower florets and cream into soup bowl before adding soup.

72. Chervil Soup

1/2 tbsp. vegetable fat
A little onion
1 medium potato, diced
1/2 tbsp. flour
2 cups vegetable stock
1 pinch of salt
1 tbsp. chervil, chopped
1 tbsp. cream*

Sauté onion in melted fat. Add diced potato and sauté. Sprinkle flour over mixture. Add stock and salt; simmer 1/2 hour and strain. Put chervil and cream into soup bowl and pour soup over them.

73. Spring Vegetable Soup

1/2 tbsp. vegetable fat
1 tbsp. flour
2 cups water or vegetable stock
1 pinch of salt
A little onion
1 tbsp. tender carrots
Spinach leaves
6 tbsp. milk*
1 tbsp. cream*
Season with: Rosemary, sorrel, nettle or
    dandelion leaves.

Melt fat. Sauté flour slightly. Add stock and salt and simmer 1/2 hour. Cut onion and vegetables fine, add to soup, let stand for a few minutes. Add milk. Put cream into soup bowl and add soup.

74. Cream of Leek Soup

1/2 tbsp. vegetable fat
1/4 leek, sliced coarsely
1-1/2 tbsp. flour
2-1/2 cups vegetable stock
1 pinch salt
1 tbsp. cream*
1 egg yolk may be added*
Season with: Brewer's yeast extract, nutmeg.

Sauté leek until it is limp. Sprinkle with flour. Add stock and salt and simmer for 1/2-3/4 hour. Strain. Put cream and egg yolk into soup bowl and add soup.

75. Onion Soup

1/2 tbsp. vegetable fat
1 onion, cut in strips
1 tbsp. flour

2 cups water or vegetable stock
1 pinch of salt
1 tbsp. cream*
Season with: Brewer's yeast extract, basil,
    nutmeg.

Melt fat. Sauté onion. Sprinkle flour over onion and sauté a little longer. Add stock and salt and simmer for 1/2 hour. Put cream into soup bowl before adding soup. Soup may be strained, if desired.

76. Potato Soup with Leek

1/2 tbsp. vegetable fat
1/2 leek, cut in fine strips
1/2 tbsp. flour
2 cups vegetable stock
1 medium potato, diced
1 pinch of salt
1 tbsp. cream*
Season with: Brewer's yeast extract, basil,
    marjoram.

Sauté leeks in fat until limp. Sprinkle flour over leeks. Add stock, potato, and salt, and simmer until tender. Put cream into soup bowl before adding soup.

77. Brown Potato Soup

1/2 tbsp. vegetable fat
1 tbsp. flour
2 cups water
1 medium potato, sliced
1 pinch of salt
1/2 tbsp. cream*
A little fresh butter or nut puree
Season with: Caraway, or marjoram.

Brown flour in saucepan. Stir in water. Add potato, salt, and cream if desired. Cook until tender. Put cheese and butter into soup bowl before adding soup.

78. Cabbage Soup with Potatoes

1/2 tbsp. vegetable fat
A little onion
1 cup collards, finely chopped
1/2 tbsp. flour
1 potato, sliced
2 cups water
1 pinch of salt
1 tbsp. cream or milk*
Season with: Dill or caraway.

Sauté onion and collards until limp. Sprinkle flour over mixture and sauté briefly. Add potato, water, and salt and simmer for 1/2 hour. Put cream into soup bowl before adding soup.

79. Bean Soup

1/2 tbsp. vegetable fat
1/2 clove of garlic
2 oz. beans, French cut
A little water
1 pinch of salt
Prepared cream soup
Season with: Marjoram, thyme, savory.

Sauté garlic in melted fat. Add beans and sauté. Add water and salt and cook until beans are soft. Add to cream soup (see recipe No. 59).

80. Pea Soup

2 oz. dried yellow (split) peas
1-1/8 cups of water
1 small potato
1-1/8 cups vegetable stock
1/2 tbsp. vegetable fat
A little onion

2 tbsp. chopped leek
1 small carrot
1 piece celery
1/2 tbsp. flour if desired
1 pinch of salt
1 tbsp. cream*
1 tbsp. croutons
Season with: Parsley, chives.

Soak peas for 12 hours in the water. Simmer potato with soaked peas in the soaking water until tender (about 1-1/2 hours). Strain. Sauté finely cut vegetables in fat, sprinkle with flour and add strained broth, stirring until smooth. Simmer 20 minutes longer. Put cream and croutons into soup bowl before adding soup.

81. Minestrone

1/2 tbsp. vegetable fat
A little onion
2 tbsp. leek
A few celery stalks
Swiss chard
3 cups water or vegetable stock
2 tomatoes or 1 tsp. tomato puree
1 tbsp. rosemary or thyme
1/2 clove of garlic
1/2 oz. noodles or rice
1 pinch of salt
1 tsp. butter or nut puree
Season with: Basil, parsley, chives.

Melt fat. Sauté onion in fat. Slice vegetables very fine and add slowly. Add water, seasoning, and herbs, season and simmer for 1/2 hour. Add garlic and noodles. Cook for 15-20 minutes. Add butter for flavor.

Vegetables
(preferably organically grown)

82. Spinach, Chopped

Remove thick stems from spinach and wash leaves thoroughly.

> 1/2 pint vegetable stock
> 7 oz. spinach
> 1/2 tbsp. vegetable fat
> A little onion, chopped
> Some garlic
> 1 tbsp. flour
> Spinach water
> 1 pinch of salt
> 1 cup raw spinach
> Season with: Peppermint leaves, sage, fresh
>   butter.

Bring stock to a boil. Dip spinach leaves in boiling water to scald. Chop or shred. Sauté in melted fat. Add liquid, simmer 1/4 hour. Add spinach and heat. Add remaining ingredients. Cut or shred raw spinach very fine and add just before serving.

83. Spinach, Whole Leaf

Remove thick stems of spinach, and wash leaves thoroughly and drain.

> 1/2 tbsp. vegetable fat
> Some chopped onion
> 10-1/2 oz. spinach
> 1 tbsp. pine nuts
> 1 tbsp. raisins
> Vegetable stock to taste
> 1 pinch of salt
> Season with: Peppermint leaves, sage, parsley.

Sauté onion in melted fat until golden brown. Add spinach to the onion with salt and simmer until soft, uncovered. Add pine nuts, raisins, stock if needed. Sprinkle with melted butter if desired.

84. Lettuce

1 head of lettuce
1 quart of water
1/2 tbsp. vegetable fat
6 tbsp. vegetable stock
1 pinch of salt
2 tbsp. cream*

Halve lettuce after washing. Semi-boil, fold, and place in a baking dish. Sauté onion in fat until golden brown and pour over lettuce. Add stock and salt and cook in oven about 30-40 minutes. Pour cream over vegetables 5 minutes before serving.

85. Endive

1 large endive head

Prepare like lettuce.

86. Chicory

2 chicory, prepared
1/2 tbsp. vegetable fat
2 tbsp. milk or cream*
1 tbsp. vegetable stock
1 pinch of salt
Some butter or nut puree
Season with: Onion, marjoram, thyme, apples.

Make cross incision in chicory stalks. Heat fat and add chicory in layers. Add milk and stock to vegetables, and simmer covered over a small flame for 1/2 hour. Pour butter over chicory before serving.

87. Swiss Chard

3 Swiss chard stalks, prepared
1/2 tbsp. vegetable fat
1/2 onion, chopped
3 tbsp. vegetable stock
Lemon juice or 1 tsp. almond puree
1 pinch of salt
Béchamel Sauce (recipe No. 177)*
Season with: Tarragon, bay leaf, lemon, clove,
    onion, parsley, and chives.

Cut chard stalks into 1" long slices. Melt fat and sauté onion and chard. Add stock and lemon juice and simmer covered, on small flame, until soft, 1/2 to 3/4 hour until done. Add Béchamel sauce and mix with vegetables.

88. Swiss Chard or Mock Asparagus

3-4 Swiss chard stalks, prepared
1/2 tbsp. vegetable fat
1/2 small onion, chopped
Lemon juice
6 tbsp. vegetable stock
Season with: Tarragon, bay leaf, cloves,
    parsley, chives.

Cut Swiss chard into 3" long slices and place in pan. Sauté onions in fat and pour over vegetables. Add lemon juice and simmer over small flame until tender (1/2-3/4 hour). Serve "asparagus" on platter. Serve with Rémoulade Sauce.

89. Celery Stalks

3-4 celery stalks, washed
1/2 tbsp. vegetable fat
1/2 onion, chopped

1 small apple, finely sliced
6 tbsp. vegetable stock
1 pinch of salt
1 tsp. almond puree
Season with: Celery leaves, brewer's yeast
    extract.

Sauté onion in fat. Cut celery in 3" strips and place in pan, and sauté. Add apple, stock, salt, and puree. Simmer 1/2-3/4 hour until tender.

90. Fennel

1 large or 2 small fennel
1/2 tbsp. vegetable fat
1/2 onion, chopped
6 tbsp. vegetable stock
1 pinch of salt
1 tsp. almond puree

Halve washed fennel and place in pan. Sauté onion in fat and pour over fennel. Add stock and salt. Simmer till tender. Bring puree to a boil and pour over prepared fennel before serving.

91. Spanish Artichoke

2-3 artichokes
1/2 tbsp. vegetable oil
Lemon juice
6 tbsp. vegetable stock
1 pinch of salt
Season with: Rosemary, cloves.

Prepare artichokes, slice into 3-1/2" pieces, and place in pan. Pour over vegetables, oil, juice, salt, and stock. Simmer 3/4 to 1 hour until tender. Serve on platter, sprinkle with cheese and glaze with melted nut puree or 1 tsp. almond puree.

92. Carrots, Steamed

1 tbsp. vegetable fat
1/2 small onion
Pinch of sugar and salt
3-4 carrots cut in slices or sticks
6 tbsp. vegetable stock
1 tsp. almond puree
Season with: Parsley, marjoram, some bay,
    thyme, rosemary.

Sauté onion in fat. Add sugar and salt. Add carrots and simmer in stock 1/2-3/4 hour until tender. Add purée.

93. Carrots in Sauce, I

1/4 tbsp. vegetable fat
3-4 carrots cut in small slices
1/2 tbsp. butter or nut puree
1/2 tbsp. flour
1 pinch of salt
3 tbsp. milk*
3 tbsp. water or vegetable stock
Season with: Sugar (brown), onions (golden brown),
    parsley, rosemary, marjoram, bay leaf, thyme.

Sauté carrots until half tender. Prepare a thin sauce, add carrots and simmer for about 1/2 hour until done.

94. Carrots in Sauce, II

3/4 cup vegetable stock
3-4 carrots, thin sticks
1/2 tbsp. fresh butter or nut puree
1 level tbsp. flour
6 tbsp. milk and carrot juice
1 pinch of salt

1 tbsp. cream
Season with: Onion (golden brown), parsley,
    rosemary, marjoram, bay leaf, thyme.

Cook carrots in stock until tender. Prepare Béchamel sauce, recipe No. 177. Add cream to improve flavor. Mix sauce with finished carrots and serve.

95. Peas with Carrots

1/4 tbsp. vegetable fat
1/4 onion, chopped
3-1/2 oz. peas, shelled
6 tbsp. vegetable stock
1/4 tbsp. vegetable fat
Onion, chopped
5 oz. prepared carrots
6 tbsp. vegetable stock
1 pinch of salt
Season with: Parsley, chives, marjoram, thyme,
    rosemary.

Sauté onion in fat. Add peas, stock, seasoning. Simmer until done. Cut carrots into thin sticks, and prepare like steamed carrots, recipe No. 92. Mix finished vegetables in pan or arrange on platter, alternating peas and carrots.

96. Green Peas

1/2 tbsp. vegetable fat
1/4 onion, chopped
1/2 tbsp. sugar
1/2 lb. peas, shelled
6 tbsp. vegetable stock
1 pinch of salt
2 tsp. liquefied nut puree
Season with: Parsley, chives, marjoram, thyme,
    rosemary.

Melt fat. Sauté onion in fat. Add peas, stock, seasoning and simmer over very low heat until tender, 20 to 40 minutes, according to quality. Pour nut puree over peas to glaze.

97. Green Peas, French Style

1/2 tbsp. vegetable fat
1/2 onion
1/2 head of lettuce, cut in thin strips
5-7 oz. peas, shelled
6 tbsp. vegetable stock
1 pinch of salt
2 tsp. nut puree
1 tbsp. flour
Season with: Parsley, chives, marjoram, thyme,
    rosemary.

Melt fat. Sauté onion in fat. Add lettuce and simmer. Add peas, stock, salt and simmer over very low heat until peas are tender. Mix nut puree with flour and bring to a boil. Add to peas.

98. Green Peas with Pearl Onions

1/2 tbsp. vegetable fat
2 oz. pearl onions, prepared
6 oz. green peas, shelled
6 tbsp. vegetable stock
1 pinch of salt
Basil, chopped
Season with: Parsley, chives, marjoram, thyme,
    rosemary, fresh butter or nut puree.

Melt fat. Sauté onions in fat until golden. Add peas, stock, salt and simmer covered until peas are tender Sprinkle a little chopped basil over the peas if desired.

99. Chinese Snow Peas (Sugar Peas), Sauteed

1/2 tbsp. vegetable fat
1/2 onion, chopped
7 oz. snow peas, prepared
6 tbsp. vegetable stock
1 pinch of salt
Parsley or rosemary
Season with: Chives, marjoram, thyme; dot with
    fresh butter or nut puree.

Melt fat. Sauté onion in fat. Add peas, stock, and salt
and steam everything together in a covered pan for 1/2-1
hour. Add parsley or rosemary while cooking or sprinkle
over peas before serving.

100. Green Beans

1/2 tbsp. vegetable fat
1/2 chopped onion
Some garlic
1/2 lb. beans
Savory
Parsley
1-2 tomatoes, diced small
1 pinch of salt
Season with: caraway, marjoram, rosemary.

Melt fat. Sauté onion and garlic in fat until golden. Add
beans, savory, and parsley and sauté together. Add tomatoes and salt in place of vegetable stock, and simmer about
1 hour.

101. Celery root (Celeriac)

1/2 tbsp. vegetable fat
1/2 onion
1/2 celery root, washed
6 tbsp. vegetable stock
1 pinch of salt
1 tsp. almond puree
Season with: Lemon juice, apple, marjoram,
    nuts.

Melt fat. Sauté onion in fat. Cut celery root into small
slices and sauté with onions. Add stock and salt and simmer 1/2-3/4 hour, until celery root is tender. Add almond
puree for added flavor.

102. Celery Root (Celeriac) with Béchamel Sauce*

1 small celery root
Ingredients as above
Season with: Lemon juice, apple, marjoram, nuts,
    sugar.

Prepare as above. When finished, mix with Béchamel
Sauce, recipe No. 177, and serve.

103. Celery-Root Slices with Hollandaise Sauce

1 medium celery root, peeled and quartered
3 tbsp. milk
3 tbsp. water
1 pinch of salt
Hollandaise Sauce
Season with: Cheese, bread crumbs, and
glaze with melted butter.

Boil celeriac and salt until soft in milk and water. Cut
into slices 1/3" thick and arrange on platter. Pour Hollandaise Sauce over.

104. Viper's Grass, Sauteed

(Oyster Plant may also be prepared in this way.)

About 9 oz. viper's grass, cleaned
1/2 tbsp. vegetable fat
1/2 onion
6 tbsp. vegetable stock
1 pinch of salt
1 tsp. almond puree
Season with: Lemon juice, rosemary, bay, cloves,
    basil, celery leaves, brewer's yeast extract,
    parsley, onion, chives.

Cut viper's grass into finger-long pieces, place in pan.
Sauté onion in fat. Pour over vegetable. Add stock and
salt and simmer covered over low heat for 1 hour. Add
puree when almost cooked.

105. Red Beets

3/4 lb. beets
1/2 tbsp. vegetable fat
1/2 onion, chopped
6 tbsp. vegetable stock
Pinch of sugar and salt
Lemon juice
1/4 bay leaf
1/2 tbsp. flour
Cold water
1 tbsp. almond puree
Season with: Lemon, rosemary, caraway, lemon
    balm, nutmeg, trace of garlic or horseradish,
    parsley.

Cut tips and leaves off beets to about 2/3", wash thoroughly. Do not damage skin. Boil beets until tender (2-3
hours or about 25 minutes in pressure cooker), rinse in
cold water, peel and cut in thin slices. Melt fat and sauté
onion in it. Add vegetables, stock, sugar, salt and lemon

juice. Add bay leaf. Mix well and simmer 1/4 hour. Blend flour with a little cold water and add to beets. Add puree last.

106. Jerusalem Artichokes

9 oz. Jerusalem artichokes
1/2 tbsp. vegetable fat
1/2 onion
1 tsp. almond puree
Season with: Basil.

Cook artichokes in their skins like potatoes (recipe No. 139). Peel and cut in slices. Melt fat and sauté onion in it. Add artichokes. Continue sautéeing. Add puree for added flavor.

May also be served with Béchamel sauce, recipe No. 177, and grated cheese.*

107. Tomatoes

4-5 tomatoes
1 tbsp. oil
1/2 tbsp. vegetable fat
1/2 onion
Sugar
1 pinch of salt
A little garlic
1 tbsp. cornstarch
Season with: Rosemary, marjoram, basil, bay,
    nutmeg (chives, dill, parsley).

Scald tomatoes with boiling water and peel. (Very ripe tomatoes can be peeled without scalding.) Brown onion lightly in fat in a frying pan. Cut tomatoes in pieces, add to onions and sauté until somewhat reduced. Add sugar, garlic, salt and finish cooking. To thicken, add cornstarch near the end of cooking time. Sprinkle plenty of chopped parsley or other herbs over tomatoes before serving.

108. Tomatoes, Baked

2-3 tomatoes
1 pinch of salt
2 tsp. vegetable fat
Season with: Parsley, onions (fried and sprinkled
    over tomatoes).

Halve tomatoes and place on greased cookie sheet or in
fireproof dish. Salt. Place dab of fat on each tomato half
and bake in oven for a few minutes. If desired, some
tomatoes may be chopped in blender or finely by hand,
mixed with cream, brought to a boil and poured over the
baked tomatoes before serving*.

109. Tomatoes with Cheese Slices

2 tomatoes
1 oz. cheese
Season with: Parsley.

Halve tomatoes and place on greased cookie sheet or in
fireproof dish. Cut cheese in thin slices the size of the
tomatoes and place on tomato halves. Bake in oven until
cheese is melted.

110. Tomatoes, Stuffed

2-3 tomatoes
3 tsp. rice
1 pinch of salt
Butter or nut puree
Herbs
Vegetable stock if desired
Season with: Onion, garlic, rosemary, marjoram,
    thyme, basil, bay, nutmeg, parsley, dill, chives.

Cut tops off tomatoes, and set aside. Hollow them out.
Chop the tomato pulp and mix with 1 tsp. of uncooked rice

per tomato; season to taste with herbs. Fill tomato shells with the mixture, add a dab of butter to each, and cover with cut-off lids. Bake in the oven up to 30 minutes over high heat.

111. Zucchini (Squash)

1/2 tbsp. vegetable fat
Onion, chopped
1 tbsp. oil
10-11 oz. zucchini
2 oz. tomatoes
Small onion, chopped
1 pinch of salt
Season with: Garlic, rosemary, marjoram, thyme,
    basil, bay leaf, nutmeg, parsley, chives, dill.

Melt fat. Sauté onion in fat. Dice zucchini (in large zucchini scoop out seeds), and add to onion. Sauté. Peel and dice tomatoes. Sauté and add onion to finished zucchini or fry raw diced tomatoes with zucchini. If there is too much liquid, a little cornmeal and 1 tsp. almond puree can be added for thickening.

112. Zucchini, Baked

7 oz. zucchini (approx.)
1 pinch of salt
Flour for dipping
Oil or vegetable fat for frying

Cut zucchini in finger-length strips or 1/3" thick slices. Salt. Spread on dish, leave a few minutes and then quickly dip in flour and deep-fry in oil or vegetable fat.

113. Zucchini Chips

Like potato chips, zucchini may be cut right into hot oil or vegetable fat, and removed with a skimming ladle when golden brown; salt lightly.

114. Peppers, Green, Yellow or Red, Sauteed

Peppers are more suitable as additions to other dishes, rather than as main dishes.

    5-7 oz. peppers
    1 tbsp. oil
    1/2 onion
    1 pinch of salt
    Season with: Garlic, rosemary, marjoram, thyme,
        basil, bay leaf, nutmeg, parsley.

Cut pepper in strips and simmer in oil, with onion and salt, in covered frying pan, for 1/2 hour.

115. Peperonata

    2 oz. peppers
    4 oz. zucchini
    2 oz. eggplant
    1 tomato
    1/2 onion
    Some garlic
    1 tbsp. oil
    2 oz. potatoes
    1 pinch of salt
    Season with: Rosemary, marjoram, thyme, basil,
        bay leaf, nutmeg, parsley.

Halve peppers; remove seeds, and dice. Peel squash and eggplant and tomato and cut in fair-sized cubes. Chop onion fine and brown with garlic in oil. Simmer with vegetables. Cut potatoes in 1/3" cubes, add and simmer all together 1–1-1/2 hours. If too much liquid develops, reduce it by simmering, uncovered. Add salt.

116. Eggplant

7 oz. eggplant (approx.)
Oil for frying
1 tomato
1 pinch of salt

Cut washed eggplant in slices and fry in fair amount of oil until almost done; place in soufflé dish. Cut tomato in slices and put on top. Sprinkle with grated or sliced cheese or a little bread crumbs.* Add flakes of nut puree and bake in oven for 1/2 hour.

117. Artichokes

1 artichoke
1-1/2 pt. water
1 tbsp. lemon juice
1 pinch of salt

Cut stems off artichokes. Remove hard lower leaves and tips. Halve them and remove flower center, wash under running water and rub cut surface with lemon juice. Bring water and salt to a boil, simmer artichoke until tender, about 3/4 hour. Drain and arrange on a napkin on a warm platter. Serve with Hollandaise* Sauce or Remoulade or Vinaigrette Sauce.

118. Asparagus

1/2 bunch asparagus
1 quart water
1 pinch of salt

Wash asparagus, taking care not to break them. Boil until tender for 20-30 minutes in a long pan, with the salt. Take out with a skimming ladle and arrange on a napkin-covered platter. Serve with Vinaigrette Sauce. Glaze with grated cheese* and liquid nut puree.

119. Corn on the Cob

1-2 ears of corn
1 quart of water
1 pinch of salt

Only use ears of corn that are milky tender. Remove husks and silk. Boil corn 10-20 minutes until tender. Serve on hot platter which has been covered with a folded napkin. Serve with fresh nut puree.

120. Cauliflower

1 small cauliflower
1 quart water
1 pinch of salt
Season with: Butter sauce with tarragon and lemon— or liquefied nut puree, parsley, chives.

Remove leaves and stalk of cauliflower; cut into fairly large floret sections. Peel stem, retaining tender leaves. Soak in cold water with salt for 1 hour, then rinse thoroughly. Cook until tender, 20-30 minutes, drain. Arrange on hot deep platter.

Cauliflower which is not young and tender needs to be scalded before using.

121. Brussels Sprouts

1/2 tbsp. vegetable fat
7 oz. Brussels sprouts, cleaned
6 tbsp. vegetable stock
1 pinch of salt
Season with: Nutmeg, basil.

Sauté Brussels sprouts lightly. Add stock and simmer for 1/2 hour until tender. Add salt. Serve glazed with liquid nut puree or covered with Béchamel Sauce, recipe No. 177.

122. White Cabbage, Sautéed

1/2 tbsp. vegetable fat
1/2 onion, chopped
9 oz. young cabbage
6 tbsp. vegetable stock
1 pinch of salt
Basil or rosemary
Brewer's yeast extract if desired
Nutmeg
Caraway
Season with: Some garlic, parsley.

(Green, tough cabbage must first be scalded in water.)
Melt fat and sauté onion in it. Cut the cabbage in 3/4"
strips, add to onion, sauté until vegetables are limp; add
liquid and simmer over low heat for 1/2 hour until tender.
Add herbs and spices for flavor.

123. Cabbage, Chopped

7 oz. cabbage
1 quart water
1 tbsp. vegetable fat
1/2 chopped Zwieback
1 onion (small), chopped
Garlic
1 small tbsp. flour
6 tbsp. vegetable stock
1-2 tbsp. cream*
Brewer's yeast extract
Nutmeg
1 pinch of salt
Season with: Caraway, parsley.

Quarter cabbage, boil in salted water until tender, and
drain. Chop fine. Melt fat and sauté until golden brown,
Zwieback, onion, and garlic. Sprinkle flour over onion and

brown slightly. Add stock and simmer for 1/4 hour, then
add cabbage and heat. For added flavor, add cream, yeast,
nutmeg, and salt.

124. Savoy Cabbage

Prepared like cabbage.

125. Tart White Cabbage

1 tbsp. vegetable fat
1/2 onion
9 oz. white cabbage, shredded or cut fine
1/2 tbsp. lemon juice
1/2 tbsp. flour
3 tbsp. vegetable stock
3 tbsp. sweet cider
Caraway
1 pinch of salt
Season with: A little garlic, rosemary, nutmeg, apple,
    tomato, mushrooms.

Melt fat. Sauté onion in the fat. Add cabbage and lemon
juice and sauté together. Sprinkle flour over cabbage mixture. Add stock and cider, caraway, and salt, and simmer
covered for 1 hour.

126. Red Cabbage

1 tbsp. vegetable fat
1/2 onion, chopped
9 oz. red cabbage, finely shredded
1/2 tbsp. lemon juice
1/2 apple, cut in thin slices
1/2 tbsp. rice
6 tbsp. vegetable stock
3 tbsp. grape juice or sweet cider
1 pinch of salt
1 apple, peeled, cut in sections
A little butter or nut puree

Melt fat and saute onion in it. Add cabbage and saute together. Add lemon juice and apple. Stir in rice. Add stock and juice and salt, and simmer covered on low heat 1-1-1/2 hours until tender. Butter apple sections and bake in the oven on a cookie sheet. Use to garnish red cabbage before serving.

127. Kohlrabi with Herbs*

1 kohlrabi
1/2 tbsp. vegetable fat
1/2 onion, chopped
6 tbsp. vegetable stock
1 tbsp. tender kohlrabi leaves, chopped
1 tbsp. cream
Prepare Béchamel Sauce, recipe No. 177.

Quarter kohlrabi, then cut in thin slices. Sauté onion in melted fat and add vegetables. Add stock and simmer covered 1/2-1 hour. Add kohlrabi leaves last with the cream. Add various other chopped herbs to Béchamel Sauce and mix with finished kohlrabi.

128. Leeks, I*

7 oz. prepared leeks
1/2 tbsp. vegetable fat
6 tbsp. vegetable stock
1 tbsp. cream
A little grated cheese to taste.

Cut leeks in 4" long pieces. Melt fat and add leeks in frying pan. Add stock and cook slowly, covered. Add cream and cheese last.

129. Onions

1/2 tbsp. vegetable fat
7 oz. pearl onions
Pinch of sugar and salt
6 tbsp. vegetable stock

Melt fat. Sauté onions slowly in fat. Add stock, sugar and salt, and simmer 3/4 hour. This vegetable can be garnished with green peas or may be served with Béchamel Sauce, recipe No. 177.*

130. Chestnuts

9 oz. chestnuts
1/2 tbsp. vegetable fat
1/2 tbsp. sugar
6 tbsp. vegetable stock
1 pinch of salt
1 tbsp. cream*
Fresh butter or nut puree

Slit the chestnut shells and place in hot oven until they crack open; peel. Melt fat and brown the sugar in it. Pour stock and salt on browned sugar and add chestnuts. Cook about 1/2 hour, until liquid disappears. Pour butter, or cream and butter over chestnuts before serving.

The chestnuts can also be prepared without sugar. They are then sautéed with a chopped onion and cooked in bouillon or stock. A sliced, steamed onion is arranged on the top of the chestnuts before serving.

131. Mixed Vegetables

1 tbsp. vegetable fat
1/2 onion, chopped
2 oz. celery
2 oz. carrots
6 tbsp. vegetable stock
2 oz. cauliflower
2 oz. peas or beans
6 tbsp. vegetable stock
1 pinch of salt

Melt fat and saute onion. Cube celery and carrots and add to onions. Saute. Add stock and simmer till vegetables are tender. Cook cauliflower in a little milk and water until tender. Add peas and cook until tender, in the stock.

Salads Made with Cooked Vegetables

Carrots, celery, beets, beans, cauliflower, squash, are especially suitable for these salads.

The vegetables are boiled in vegetable stock or in water until tender and then cut into small pieces (cubes, slices, clusters). Mix with salad dressing or with diluted mayonnaise*. Cauliflower may also be covered with a Remoulade Sauce. Use onions and chopped herbs for seasoning.

132. Potato Salad

7 oz. potatoes
3 tbsp. vegetable stock, hot
1 tbsp. oil
1 tbsp. lemon juice
1/2 tbsp. cream*
1/2 tbsp. onions, chopped
1 pinch of salt
Season with: Borage, chives, parsley, lemon balm,
    marjoram, thyme, dill.

Boil potatoes in skins; peel while hot and slice. Cover with hot stock. Let potatoes stand for a while. Blend well oil, lemon juice, and cream, and mix with potatoes. Add onions and salt.

133. Potato Salad with Cucumbers

1 large potato
1/4 cucumber
1/2 tbsp. oil
1/2 tbsp. lemon juice
1 pinch of salt
Season with: Dill or borage, chives, parsley, onion.
    Rub dish with garlic.

Prepare potato as for potato salad. Grate cucumber on coarse grater. Mix oil and lemon juice with dressing or mayonnaise and potato salad.

134. Mixed Salad (Cooked Vegetables)

For this type of salad, use 3-4 different vegetables, boiled, sliced, or diced, and mix with salad dressing, such as carrots, celery, cauliflower, squash, zucchini, beans, beets, stir into creamed mixture and season. Serve on hot platter. ley, marjoram, thyme, dill.

135. Salade Nicoise

1 boiled potato
1 small tomato
Radishes
Several cucumber slices
1 tbsp. oil
1/2 tbsp. lemon juice
Onion, garlic if desired
1 pinch of salt
Herbs
Several lettuce leaves
Season with: Parsley, chives or dill, lemon balm, borage.

Slice potato. Prepare salad dressing (oil, lemon juice, onion, garlic, herbs) and mix with vegetables. Mix with salad before serving. May also be prepared with mayonnaise*.

136. Rice Salad

2 oz. rice
3/4 cup water
1 tbsp. oil
1/2 tbsp. lemon juice
1 pinch of salt
1/2 tbsp. onion, chopped
1/2 tomato, diced
Lettuce leaves
Season with: Chives, parsley or basil.

Boil rice until done, rinse, and let cool. Blend oil and lemon juice; mix with onion and add to rice. Mix tomatoes in gently. Arrange finished salad on lettuce leaves, serve in shells for special occasions.

137. Celery-Root (Celeriac) Salad with Soy Sauce

1/2 small celery root (Celeriac), raw
1/2-1 tbsp. lemon juice
2 walnuts, coarsely chopped
1/4 apple, grated, if desired
1 pinch of salt
1 tbsp. soy sauce

Cut celery root into matchstick-thin strips, or grate. Add lemon juice and mix. Add walnuts, apple, and salt. Add soy sauce and mix carefully.

138. Vegetable Mold (Aspic)

1 cup vegetable stock, warm
1/2 tsp. Agar-Agar†, powdered
Several drops lemon juice
Salt, a pinch
Brewer's yeast extract
Fresh cucumbers
Diced tomatoes
Cauliflower clusters, boiled
Green peas, boiled
Beans, boiled

Dissolve Agar-Agar in warm stock; heat slowly, until Agar-Agar is completely dissolved. For seasoning, add lemon juice, brewer's yeast, and salt. Put small amount of aspic in rinsed bowls or molds; set aside to get firm in a cool spot. Arrange vegetable slices over aspic, allow to set, etc., adding vegetables and aspic alternately, until mold is full. Unmold and use to garnish salad platters.

† Agar-Agar is obtainable in powder form at health-food stores. It is a vegetable gelatin made from seaweed.

Potato Dishes

139. Jacket Potatoes

White or red potatoes are especially suitable.

3-4 small potatoes
water
1 pinch of salt

Scrub potatoes with a vegetable brush, and rinse. Use pan with perforated insert or a wire basket, fill with water up to insert, put in potatoes with salt, cover and steam 30-40 minutes; or in pressure cooker according to manufacturer's instructions.

140. Baked Potatoes

3-4 small potatoes
1 tbsp. oil
Margarine
Nut puree

Scrub potatoes with a vegetable brush; rinse. Make 3 or 4 small cuts in skins on top, dab with oil, and bake on greased cookie sheet 30-40 minutes at medium heat. Place a dab of nut puree on each potato before serving.

141. Potatoes with Cottage Cheese

3-4 small potatoes
1 tbsp. oil
Stuffing:
    2 oz. cottage cheese
    1-2 tbsp. milk or cream
    Chives or caraway or marjoram
    1 pinch of salt

Make a cut across tops of potatoes and prepare like

baked potatoes. Mix cottage cheese and milk or cream with chives, salt, etc. until smooth. Add other ingredients. Squeeze filling over cut in the baked potatoes through a pastry bag. This stuffing can also be served with baked potatoes.

142. Potatoes with Caraway Seeds

2-3 medium potatoes (oblong, thin)
1 tsp. caraway seeds
Pinch of salt

Brush and rinse potatoes. Halve them lengthwise. Mix together caraway and salt, dip the cut side of the potatoes into the mixture. Place on greased cookie sheet, cut side down. Dab with oil and bake at medium heat for 3/4 hour.

143. Bouillon Potatoes

9 oz. potatoes
6-12 tbsp. vegetable stock
1 pinch of salt
2 tsp. butter or nut puree
Season with: Rosemary, some thyme, bay leaf.

Wash potatoes, peel, halve or cut in pieces and boil until soft in stock. Add salt. Dot potatoes with butter before serving.

144. Parsley Potatoes

9 oz. potatoes, peeled
A little water
1 pinch of salt
1 tbsp. fresh butter or nut puree
1 tbsp. parsley, chopped

Quarter potatoes lengthwise. Salt. Steam potatoes in a wire basket. Set in a pan of boiling water or a steamer. Melt butter, mix with parsley, add to potatoes and serve.

145. Potatoes with Cream*

7 oz. potatoes, peeled
1/2 tbsp. butter
6 tbsp. vegetable stock
1 pinch of salt
3 tbsp. cream or milk
Parsley
Season with: Thyme, small clove, nutmeg, brewer's
    yeast extract, lightly browned onion.

Slice potatoes. Sauté in the butter. Add stock and cook in stock until the potatoes are tender. Add cream and salt before serving. Sprinkle potatoes with parsley.

146. Potatoes with Tomatoes

1/2 tbsp. vegetable fat
1/2 small onion
7 oz. potatoes
6 tbsp. vegetable stock
1 small tomato
1 pinch of salt
1 tbsp. cream*
Season with: Marjoram or rosemary or thyme,
    maybe nutmeg.

Sauté onion in fat until it is light brown. Add peeled, sliced potatoes, vegetable stock, and salt. Parboil. Peel tomato, cut in slices and add to potatoes cooking until done. Add cream before serving.

147. Potato Mousse

4 potatoes
Water
Butter
Season with: dried tomatoes, finely cut and sprinkled
    over the dish; golden onion rings.

Wash, peel, and cut potatoes. Soft boil in very little water. Force through a sieve onto a warm platter. Pour melted butter over potatoes.

148. Mashed Potatoes*

4 potatoes
Water
2 tsp. butter
6 tbsp. milk
Nutmeg
1 tbsp. cream if desired
1 pinch of salt
Season with: Finely chopped marjoram, golden brown
    onion rings, garlic, finely chopped caraway seed,
    finely grated dried tomatoes.

Peel potatoes, cut in pieces, and steam or boil in a little water until done. Add salt. Squeeze through potato press (or sieve, or mash). Warm butter and milk; add potatoes, stir into cream mixture and season. Serve on hot platter. Dip knife in hot water to decorate mashed potatoes.

149. Potato Balls*

4 potatoes
6 tbsp. milk
2 tsp. butter or nut puree
1 pinch of salt
2 tsp. butter or nut puree
Season with: Nutmeg.

Prepare potatoes like mashed potatoes. Melt butter. Dip small scoop in melted butter. Scoop out balls of potato and place in a hot pan. Put butter on top of potatoes.

150. Stewed Potatoes

2 sm. potatoes, peeled
A little water
1 pinch of salt
6 tbsp. vegetable stock
1/2 tbsp. vegetable fat, liquid
1-2 tbsp. cream* or nut puree
Season with: Small amount of cloves, bay leaf,
    nutmeg, thyme.

Halve and steam potatoes until partially done. Place in a baking dish, cut sides down. Pour vegetable stock and salt over potatoes and bake in oven until vegetable stock is absorbed. Pour fat over mixture and return to oven until slightly browned, cut sides up. Serve potatoes with cut side up and sprinkle with chopped parsley.

151. Princess Potatoes*

3 potatoes
A little water
1 tbsp. grated cheese or cottage cheese
1/2 tbsp. vegetable fat
6 tbsp. milk
1 egg
2 tbsp. milk
1 tbsp. cream or milk
Dabs of butter
Season with: Nutmeg, marjoram, finely chopped.

Steam-boil potatoes, peel, and cut in thick slices. Place into a baking dish and sprinkle with cheese. Pour melted fat and milk over potatoes; bake in oven for 10 min. Beat eggs with a whisk, add milk and cream and pour over all. Put dabs of butter on top of mixture and bake in oven 10-15 minutes.

152. Lyonnaise Potatoes

1/2 tbsp. vegetable fat
1/2 tbsp. oil
3 small potatoes, peeled
1 small onion, cut in strips
1 pinch of salt

Melt fat and heat oil. Cut potatoes in slices and sauté until partly done in hot fat. Add onions, and salt, and finish cooking until tender.

153. Potato Sticks (Fried)

3 large potatoes
1/2 tbsp. oil
1 pinch of salt
Season with: Some nutmeg and rosemary.

Peel potatoes and cut them into sticks; dry in a towel. Heat oil and add potatoes. Fry for a short time covered and then for about 1/2 hour uncovered.

154. Potato Slices with Spinach

1 large potato, peeled
6 tbsp. vegetable stock
1 pinch of salt
3-1/2 oz. spinach
1 tbsp. cheese, grated*
A little butter or nut puree
Season with: Browned onion, a little garlic, parsley, chives, perhaps peppermint or sage, nutmeg.

Cut potatoes lengthwise in 1/3" slices. Boil potatoes carefully until soft and place on buttered cookie sheet. Prepare spinach as in recipe No. 83. Place on top of potatoes. Sprinkle cheese over all. Dab butter on top and bake briefly in oven.

155. Potatoes with Kale (Meal-in-One)

1/2 tbsp. vegetable fat
1 tbsp. chopped onion
3-1/2 oz. kale, cut small
2 small potatoes, diced
Melted butter or nut puree
Season with: Finely chopped caraway seed,
    marjoram, nutmeg, basil.

Melt fat and sauté onion in it. Add kale and sauté. Add potatoes and simmer for 1/2-3/4 hour. Pour butter or nut puree over potatoes before serving.

Rice, Cereal, and Pasta

(Use brown rice or partially hulled rice.)

156. Japanese Rice

1/2 tbsp. vegetable fat
3 oz. rice
1/2-3/4 cup vegetable stock
    or celery water
1 pinch of salt
2 tsp. butter or nut puree
Season with: Small peeled onion which has been stuck
    with cloves holding a bay leaf and boiled with the
    rice.

Melt fat. Sauté rice in fat. Add stock and salt and simmer, covered, 15 minutes. Rice should remain granular; let cool. Heat butter, add rice and sauté until hot.

157. Risotto

1/2 tbsp. vegetable fat
1 tbsp. chopped onion
3 oz. rice
3/4 cup vegetable stock or water
1 pinch of salt
2 tsp. fresh butter or nut puree
2/3 oz. Parmesan cheese, grated
Season with: Mushrooms, finely chopped; fresh
    herbs to taste, rosemary.

Melt fat. Sauté rice with onion until it becomes transparent. Add hot stock and salt and simmer 15 to 20 minutes. Mix butter and cheese in with a fork before serving.

158. Saffron Rice

Prepare like risotto. Dissolve a pinch of saffron powder in a little bouillon and add.
Season with: Mushrooms, finely chopped, fresh herbs to taste, rosemary.

159. Rice Creole with Vegetables

1/2 tbsp. vegetable fat
2 tbsp. vegetables, very finely diced
    (leek, celery, carrots)
3 oz. rice
1 pinch of salt
3/4 cup vegetable stock
Season with: Bay leaf, clove, nutmeg; always use
    freshly chopped herbs to taste.

Melt fat, sauté all ingredients together, except stock. Add hot stock and simmer 15 to 20 minutes.

160. Tomato Rice

1/2 tbsp. vegetable fat
1 tbsp. onion, chopped
A little garlic
3 oz. rice
1 large tomato
6 tbsp. vegetable stock (approx.)
1 pinch of salt
2 tsp. fresh butter, or nut puree
Season with: Rosemary, marjoram, clove, bay leaf,
    perhaps basil, nutmeg; mix a little sugar with
    tomatoes and onions.

Melt fat and sauté onion and garlic. Add rice and sauté
until transparent. Peel tomatoes and dice; add to the rice
mixture. Add salt and stock. Simmer 15-20 minutes. Mix
in butter before serving.

161. Risotto with Peppers

1 tbsp. oil
1 tbsp. onion, chopped
1/2 pepper, cut in strips
2 oz. rice
6 tbsp. vegetable stock
1 pinch of salt
Season with: Rosemary, marjoram, clove, bay leaf,
    perhaps basil, nutmeg.

If peppers are too sharp, they may be cut and soaked in
cold water for an hour before cooking. Heat oil and sauté
onions and pepper in it. Add rice and sauté together until
the rice appears transparent. Add stock and salt and bake
in the oven for 15 minutes or simmer until done on top of
the stove.

162. Rice with Zucchini

1/2 tbsp. oil
1 tbsp. onion, chopped
5 oz. tender zucchini
1 pinch of salt
A little vegetable stock or water
3 oz. rice
9 tbsp. water or vegetable stock
2 tsp. butter or nut puree
Season with: Brewer's yeast extract, freshly
    chopped dill.

Heat oil and sauté onion. Dice zucchini, add and sauté
with onions for 10 minutes. Add part of stock and rice,
gradually adding more liquid until risotto is formed. Add
butter last.

163. Rice with Green Peas

1/2 tbsp. butter or oil
Some onion, chopped
A little sugar and salt
5 oz. green peas, shelled
3 tbsp. vegetable stock
1/2 tbsp. vegetable fat
Some onion, chopped
3 oz. rice
1/2-3/4 cup water
2 tsp. butter or nut puree
Season with: Chopped parsley, perhaps cloves.

Melt butter or heat oil. Sauté onion until golden. Add
peas and sauté lightly with onion. Add stock, then simmer
until tender. Prepare Risotto (see recipe No. 161) and add
cooked green peas to finished dish. Add butter to rice before serving.

164. Rice with Spinach

1/2 tbsp. butter or oil
Some onion, chopped
3-1/2 oz. spinach, coarsely cut
3 oz. rice
3/4 cup vegetable stock or water, hot
1 pinch of salt ·
2 tsp. fresh butter or nut puree
Season with: Nutmeg and peppermint.

Melt fat and sauté onion. Add spinach and rice to the onion and sauté. Add stock and salt to the spinach mixture, and simmer 15-20 minutes. Add butter before serving.

165. Rice Soufflé with Tomatoes

1/2 tbsp. butter or oil
2 tbsp. vegetables, diced very fine
    (leek, celery, carrots)
3 oz. rice
1/2 cup vegetable stock
1 pinch of salt
2 small tomatoes, sliced
2 tsp. butter or nut puree
Season with: Browned onions, parsley, rosemary.

Melt butter or heat oil. Sauté vegetables and rice together. Add hot stock and salt, and simmer 15-20 minutes. Place rice and tomato slices in alternate layers in buttered baking dish. Dot with butter and bake in oven for 10 minutes.

166. Semolina Pudding*

2 oz. semolina
1 tbsp. sugar
1-1/8 cups milk
3/4 cup water
Pinch of salt
2 tsp. butter or nut puree
Cinnamon

Boil water and milk together. Stir semolina and salt into the boiling liquid and simmer 15-20 minutes. Melt butter and pour over semolina before serving. Sprinkle with mixture of sugar and cinnamon.

167. Semolina Gnocchi

2 oz. semolina
1-1/8 cups milk (approx.)
Nutmeg
1 pinch salt

Bring milk to a boil. Stir semolina into boiling milk. Add salt and nutmeg. Simmer 15-20 minutes. Spread out on a board, to about 1/2" thick. Let cool. Cut into round shapes. Place odd pieces, left after rounds are cut, in a buttered soufflé dish and arrange rounds over them.

1 egg
3 tbsp. milk
2 tbsp. cream
1 tbsp. chives
1 tbsp. cheese, grated
2 tsp. butter

Beat egg together with milk and cream and pour over rounds. Sprinkle top with cheese, chives, and butter. Bake slowly in oven until firm.

168. Polenta

1/2 tbsp. oil
1-1/8 cups water
2 oz. cornmeal
Nutmeg
1 pinch of salt
1/2 tbsp. fresh butter or nut puree
1 tbsp. grated cheese*

Heat oil in saucepan. Add water and bring it to a boil.
Stir cornmeal, salt and nutmeg into the boiling liquid. Cook
at low heat for 5 minutes, stirring constantly, then simmer
1-2 hours over low heat or in a Dutch oven. Mix in butter
and cheese last. If desired, may be topped with browned
onion slices and fresh butter.

169. Milletto

1/2 tbsp. oil
1 tbsp. onion, chopped
2 oz. millet
9 tbsp. vegetable stock, hot
1 pinch of salt
1 tsp. cheese*
2 tsp. butter or nut puree
1/2 onion cut in strips

Sauté onion in heated oil until onions are transparent.
Add millet and sauté lightly. Add stock and salt, and simmer for 20 minutes. Sprinkle butter and cheese on top
before serving. Sauté onion until brown and place on top.

170. Milletto with Vegetables

1/2 tbsp. oil
1 tbsp. onion, chopped
2 tbsp. chopped and diced vegetables (leek,
    celery, carrots) or carrots and green peas
1-1/2 oz. millet
9 tbsp. vegetable stock
1 pinch of salt
1 tbsp. cheese*, grated
2 tsp. fresh butter or nut puree
Season with: Rosemary and brewer's yeast extract.

Sauté onion in heated oil. Add vegetables and millet and sauté. Add stock and salt and simmer for 20 minutes. Sprinkle grated cheese and bits of butter over millet before serving.

171. Crushed Cereal Mash

2 tbsp. crushed cereal (wheat, oats, rye)
3 tbsp. water
1 pinch of salt
2-3 tbsp. water

Soak cereal for 12 hours in water. Add water and salt to cereal and simmer for 10 minutes or 1/2 hour in a double boiler.

172. Noodles* (Homemade, 4 servings)

7 ozs. flour (1/2 wholewheat)
2 eggs
1-2 tbsp. water
1 tbsp. oil
1 pinch of salt

Sieve flour onto a board and make a well in the center. Place other ingredients in the well and mix into a firm dough. The dough should not show air bubbles when cut. Leave for 1/2 hour. Roll out a quarter of the dough as thinly as possible (near-transparent) and set aside. Roll dough, cut in fine strips, and loosen each by hand. Place on a cloth to dry.

1 quart water
1 tbsp. salt
5-1/2 oz. noodles
4 tsp. butter or nut puree
Season with: Half a clove of garlic, chopped;
  basil and parsley steamed in butter and sprinkled
  on top.

Bring water and salt to a boil. Add noodles and boil about 15-20 minutes, strain well, and arrange in a dish. Melt butter and pour it over the noodles.

173. Spinach Noodles* (Homemade for 4 servings)

7 oz. flour (1/2 wholewheat)
3-1/2 oz. spinach, chopped raw
2 eggs
1 tbsp. water
1 tbsp. oil
Season with: Onion strips sautéed in butter or oil.

Preparation as for homemade noodles. Add spinach to the other ingredients.

174. Mini-Gnocchi

2-1/2 oz. flour (1/2 wholewheat)
1 egg
1 tbsp. salt
6 tbsp. milk and water
1 quart water
Salt
1 tbsp. cheese
2 tsp. butter
Season with: Onion strips sautéed in butter, chives,
  and parsley.

Sieve flour onto a board. Make a well in the center of the flour. Add eggs, salt, and milk-water, and mix all together. Beat until dough blisters, then set aside for at least 1 hour. Bring quart of water and salt to a boil. Gradually, force dough through a sieve with large perforations into the boiling water. Simmer until Mini-Gnocchi rise to the surface. Remove them with a slotted spoon and arrange on a hot platter. Sprinkle cheese over top. Melt butter and pour on top.

When the Mini-Gnocchi are cold, they can be rinsed with clear, hot water or be fried in a frying pan. Instead of rubbing the dough through a sieve, it may be placed on a damp wooden board and cut into fine strips which are dropped into the boiling water.

175. Soya Mini-Gnocchi

2-1/4 oz. wholewheat flour
2/3 oz. soy flour
6 tbsp. water
Season with: Onion strips sautéed in oil, chives
    and parsley, or tomatoes.

Prepare as for Mini-Gnocchi (recipe No. 174). The Mini-Gnocchi may be cooked in vegetable stock and served immediately on a hot platter.

176. Spinach or Tomato Mini-Gnocchi

2-1/2 oz. flour (1/3 wholewheat)
1 egg
6 tbsp. milk-water
1 handful spinach, raw, chopped or 1 tsp.
    tomato puree
1 quart water
1 tbsp. salt
Season with: Onion strips sautéed in oil, chives
    and parsley, or tomatoes.

Mix and work up into smooth Gnocchi dough (recipe No. 174), and set aside for 1 hour. Prepare as in Mini-Gnocchi recipe No. 174.

Dressings

177. Béchamel Sauce*

1/2 tbsp. butter
1 tbsp. flour
3 tbsp. milk
3 tbsp. vegetable stock or water
Season with: Nutmeg.

Melt butter, sieve in flour, and sauté lightly. Add the liquid slowly, stirring steadily and simmer for 20 minutes.

178. Herb Sauce*

Béchamel Sauce, prepare as recipe No. 177.
Thicken with egg yolk if desired.
Season with: Parsley, rosemary, chervil, basil, tarragon, etc.

179. Tomato Sauce, I

1/2 tbsp. oil
1 tbsp. onion
Some garlic
2 tbsp. carrots, celery, leek
2 small tomatoes
1 pinch of salt
Some flour
9 tbsp. vegetable stock or water
A little liquid nut puree
Pinch of sugar
Season with: Bay leaf, rosemary, thyme.

Melt fat and sauté onion and garlic. Cut up vegetables coarsely, and sauté well with onion. Cut tomatoes in pieces and add to vegetable mixture. Sauté until the liquid disappears. Sprinkle flour over the vegetables. Add stock, simmer for 1/2 hour, and strain. Add nut puree and sugar for flavor.

180. Tomato Sauce, II

3 tomatoes
1 tbsp. cream* or some nut puree
Season with: Chives, basil.

Cut tomatoes in pieces, sauté until soft, and strain. Add cream for flavor.

181. Tomato Sauce, III

1/2 tbsp. oil
1/2 small onion, chopped
2 tomatoes, peeled
Season with: Thyme, lemon juice, sugar.

Sauté onion in hot oil. Dice tomatoes and sauté until tender.

182. Onion Sauce

1/2 tbsp. oil or butter
1 small onion, cut in strips
6 tbsp. vegetable stock
1 tbsp. flour
1 pinch of salt
Butter or nut puree
Season with: Nutmeg, brewer's yeast extract.

Heat fat and sauté onion until golden brown. Add flour and sauté till flour is light brown. Add stock and salt and simmer for 20 minutes. Strain finished sauce if desired. Add butter to improve flavor.

183. Horseradish Sauce*

Béchamel, prepared as in recipe No. 177.
1/3 oz. horseradish

Add finely grated horseradish to finished sauce and cook for 5 more minutes.

184. Brown Sauce

1/2 tbsp. oil
1 tbsp. flour
6 tbsp. vegetable stock
1 pinch of salt
1 tbsp. cream*
Season with: Powdered clove, lemon juice, nutmeg.

Heat oil. Brown flour in oil, and let cool. Add stock and salt and simmer for 20 minutes. Add cream for flavor if desired.

185. Mushroom Sauce

1/2 tbsp. butter
1 tbsp. onion, chopped
3-1/2 oz. fresh mushrooms
1/2 tbsp. flour
3 tbsp. vegetable stock
1 pinch of salt
Some lemon juice
1 tbsp. cream*
1 egg yolk*
Season with: Nutmeg, parsley, brewer's yeast extract.

Melt butter and saute onion. Cut mushrooms in fine slices and add to onion. Saute 1/4 hour, covered. Sprinkle flour on top. Add stock, salt and lemon juice and simmer for 10 minutes or until done. Add cream and egg yolk to improve flavor.

186. Green Pepper Sauce

1/2 tbsp. oil
1 tbsp. onion, chopped
1 tbsp. green peppers, cut in fine strips
1 tbsp. flour
6 tbsp. vegetable stock
1 pinch of salt
1 tbsp. cream* if desired
Season with: Bay leaf

Melt fat and sauté onion and peppers. Sprinkle flour over top. Add stock, salt, and bay leaf, and cook 20 minutes. Add cream to improve flavor.

187. Mayonnaise, I (for 4 servings*)

1 egg yolk
1 tbsp. lemon juice
3/4 cup oil
Season with: Brewer's yeast extract, chopped onions, and herbs.

Add a few drops of lemon juice to egg yolk and stir thoroughly. Add droplets of oil while beating steadily with an egg whisk. If the mayonnaise gets too thick, thin with a little lemon juice. Season.

188. Mayonnaise, II (for 4 servings*)

1 egg yolk
1 tbsp. lemon juice
6-9 tbsp. oil
6 tbsp. vegetable stock or water
1 level tbsp. flour
Season with: As above.

Prepare as for mayonnaise I. Stir vegetable stock and flour until smooth and bring to boil, let cool. Blend this rather thick sauce slowly into finished mayonnaise.

189. Mayonnaise without Animal Protein
(for 4 servings)

2 level tbsp. soy flour
6 tbsp. water
3/4 cup oil
4 tbsp. lemon juice
Season with: As above.

Mix flour and water into a smooth paste. Add oil and lemon juice alternately, beating steadily with egg whisk.

Sandwiches

Sandwiches are generally popular, either as an appetizer or for supper in summer; also for packed lunches and snacks. The various spreads and ingredients can be used in many different ways. The prettier and fresher the sandwiches look, the more appetizing they are. The diet bread should be at least day-old to facilitate cutting it into thin slices.

Basic Spreads

(For strict diets, spread only with nut puree and fill with raw foods):

4 tsp. cottage cheese
1 tsp. butter
Brewer's yeast extract
1 tbsp. cream
Chives, herbs, or caraway seeds

Beat cottage cheese and softened butter until creamy. Add yeast extract and cream, and blend in. Add herbs.

Or: Herb butter with dill or borage
Cream or milk

Mix together.

Garnishes:

The sandwiches can be decorated as follows:

With raw carrots, grated or sliced, celery or celeriac
With tomatoes, fresh cucumbers, radishes, watercress,
   onion rings, walnuts, parsley, chives, etc.

Sweets and Desserts
These recipes are for 4 servings.

(Where possible use honey to taste, fruit concentrate (or
pulp), and organic maple syrup instead of sugar.)

190. Sugar Syrup

2-3-1/2 oz. brown, raw, granulated sugar
1-1/2 cups water or
3/4 cup water and 3/4 cup grape juice
1-1/2 lbs. apricots, peaches, plums or green-
   gage plums

Stir sugar into water or juice. Bring to boil together. Remove pits from fruit, halve the fruit and boil in syrup for a
short time. Cool and arrange on serving dish.

191. Strawberries with Lemon Juice

1-1/4 lbs. strawberries, cleaned
1/2 lemon
Fruit concentrate or
2-3 tbsp. raw sugar
Halve large strawberries, add sweetener, lemon juice.

192. Fruit Salad

3-1/2 oz. brown, raw or granulated sugar
6 tbsp. water or
6-12 tbsp. grape juice or sweet cider

1-2 tbsp. lemon juice
1-1/4 lbs. apricots
    peaches
    melons
    apples
    pears (soft kinds)
    red cherries, pitted
    all types of berries

Bring sugar and water or juice to a boil and let cool. Add lemon juice. Select and combine fruit according to season. Cut fruit in thin slices and add to finished syrup.

193. Stuffed Melons

2 small melons
Fruit salad, recipe No. 192

Halve, hollow out and fill with fruit salad.

194. Fruit Jelly

1 cup water or grape juice
3 oz. sugar or fruit concentrate
2 tsp. Agar-Agar, powdered*

2-1/2 cups fruit juice (oranges, berries)
Whipped cream, if desired

Blend liquids and sweetener well with Agar-Agar and heat over low flame, stirring constantly until Agar-Agar is completely dissolved. Mix fruit juice with Agar-Agar and immediately fill in glasses or coupes. Decorate with whipped cream to taste.

---

* Agar-agar is a vegetable gelatine which can be bought in powder form and is used in place of gelatine in vegetables and fruits. sauces and puddings, etc.

195. Applesauce

1-1/2 lbs. apples
3/4 cup water or sweet cider
3-3-1/2 oz. raw, brown, or granulated sugar
Cinnamon
Lemon peel

Remove stems and flower end, cut in pieces, cook in water or juice until soft. Strain. Add sweetener, cinnamon, lemon peel, and mix.

196. Stewed Apples

1-1/2 lbs. apples
3/4-1-1/2 cups of water or sweet cider
3-1/2 oz. sugar, or honey to taste
1 lemon peel, grated
Cinnamon

Peel, remove cores, and slice. Bring liquid to a boil; add sugar and apples and cook until tender.

197. Apples, Halved

1-1/2 lbs. apples
1 pint water or sweet cider
5-1/2 oz. sugar or honey to taste
1/4 stick cinnamon
Quince, raspberry or currant jelly

Peel apples, core, halve, and hollow out. Bring juice, sweetener, and cinnamon, to a boil. Add apples gradually and cook slowly until tender. Take out with a slotted spoon and arrange on a flat platter, cut sides up. Fill the apple halves with jelly.

198. Blueberry Pudding

2 lbs. blueberries
7 oz. raw, brown sugar, or maple syrup
3/4 cup water
1 tbsp. flour
2 tbsp. water
2 tbsp. oil
2/3 oz. small bread cubes

Wash and clean berries. Cook 5-10 minutes in sweetener with water. Blend flour and water. Add to berries, bring to a boil. Place in serving dishes. Toast or fry bread cubes in butter and put on top to garnish.

199. Stewed Rhubarb

2 lbs. rhubarb
5-1/2-7 oz. raw or brown sugar
6 tbsp. water
6 tbsp. cornstarch if desired

Wash fruit and dice. Add water and sugar and boil briefly until soft. Take rhubarb out with a slotted spoon and arrange on platter. Boil juice until it thickens or mix with a little cornstarch, boil, and pour over rhubarb.

200. Strawberry Coupe

1 lb. strawberries
3-1/2 oz. raw sugar or fruit concentrate
3/4 cup cream*

Clean berries and strain through wire sieve or blend. Add sugar, and fold berries carefully into whipped cream. Decorate with whole berries.

Other fruit can also be prepared in this way.

201. Fruit Coupe

1/2 lb. fruit (pears, apricots, peaches and berries)
3/4 cup water
2-3 tsp. raw sugar or fruit concentrate
1/2 portion vanilla creme, recipe No. 204
6 tbsp. whipped cream*

Stew fruit with sweetener in water. Place scoops of vanilla creme over prepared fruit. Decorate with whipped cream.

202. Stuffed Apples

4 large or 8 small apples
4 tbsp. hazelnuts, ground
2 tbsp. white raisins
4 tbsp. cream* or almond puree
3 tbsp. raw sugar or fruit concentrate
1 lemon peel, grated
2 tsp. butter or nut puree
6-12 tbsp. cider

Remove cores and make cut around skin. Combine nuts, raisins, cream, sugar and lemon. Fill apples with mixture and place in a baking dish. Sprinkle butter and sugar over apples and add cider to 1/3" level. Bake in oven for 20-30 minutes.

203. Apple Hedgehog with Vanilla Creme

1-1/2 lbs. apples
1-1/8 cups of milk
1/2 stick of vanilla bean or 1 tsp. vanilla extract
1 tbsp. raw sugar
1 tsp. cornstarch
1 egg
6 tbsp. cream
1-1/2 oz. almonds

Prepare as for recipe No. 198 (halved apples). Prepare vanilla creme, recipe No. 204. Beat cream until stiff and fold into cooled creme. Blanch almonds. Peel, cut in thin "pegs" and lightly brown in oven. Arrange the apple halves with the cut sides down in a mound on a flat platter, stick with almond pegs (for hedgehog). Pour vanilla creme over apples.

204. Vanilla Creme*

    1-1/2 pt. milk
    1 vanilla bean or 1 tsp. extract
    1 tsp. cornstarch
    3 tbsp. milk
    3 eggs
    2-3-1/2 oz. raw or brown sugar

Bring milk and vanilla to a boil. Mix cornstarch with cold milk and add to the boiling milk; bring back to a boil briefly. Beat eggs and sugar together. Stir, add a little boiling milk, return mixture to pan, always stirring; heat almost to boiling point.

205. Strawberry or Raspberry Whip*

    3/4 lb. berries
    1/2 pt. milk
    1 tsp. cornstarch
    1 tbsp. milk
    1 egg
    2-3 tbsp. sugar or fruit concentrate
    1/2—3/4 cup cream

Clean berries and hull. Strain or mash in blender. Prepare as for vanilla creme, recipe No. 204; let cool. Mix with berries. Beat cream until stiff and fold in, or use for decorating before serving.

206. Rhubarb Whip*

14 oz. rhubarb
3–3-1/2 oz. raw sugar
1/2 pt. milk
1/2 stick vanilla bean
1 tsp. cornstarch
1 tbsp. milk
1 egg
1 tbsp. sugar
1/2-3/4 cup cream

Wash and dice rhubarb; cook until soft, and blend or strain. Prepare Vanilla Creme, recipe No. 204; cool, and mix with rhubarb. Beat cream until stiff and fold into creme or use to garnish.

207. Apricot Whip*

Prepare like Rhubarb Whip (adding 1 tsp. lemon juice).

208. Orange Whip*

Prepare like Lemon Whip, recipe No. 210.

209. Orange Whip (Not Cooked)*

1 piece orange peel
6 tbsp. water
1 small tsp. Agar-Agar, powdered
3/4 cup orange juice
1 tsp. lemon juice
5-6 tbsp. raw sugar
2 eggs
6-12 tbsp. cream

Mix orange peel, water and Agar-Agar thoroughly. Heat slowly over low heat until Agar-Agar is completely dissolved. Stir in juice and mix with dissolved Agar-Agar.

Beat eggs and sugar until creamy, and fold in fruit whip. Beat cream until stiff and fold in gently. Arrange, and let set for about 1 hour.

210. Lemon Whip*

1-1/2 pt. milk
1-2 lemons
1 tbsp. cornstarch
3 tbsp. milk
3 eggs
3-1/2-5-1/2 oz. raw sugar
6-12 tbsp. cream, whipped

Peel lemons and boil up peel in the milk. Mix cornstarch with cold milk. Add to boiling milk, and boil up briefly. Beat eggs and sugar, add a little hot milk, keep stirring and return to pan, bringing to near-boil. Cool. Strain cooled whip, add a few spoonfuls of lemon juice and mix with whipped cream.

210-A. Lemon Whip (prepared uncooked)*

1 piece of lemon peel
9 tbsp. water
1 small tsp. Agar-Agar, powdered
3-4 tbsp. lemon juice
5-6 tbsp. raw sugar or fruit concentrate
2 eggs
6-12 tbsp. cream, whipped

Prepare like orange whip, recipe No. 209.

211. Orange Gelatine Molds

1-1/8 cups orange juice
1 tsp. Agar-Agar, powdered
1 tbsp. raw sugar or fruit concentrate
3/4 cup orange juice

Mix well Agar-Agar and orange juice with sugar. Heat over low heat, stirring constantly (do not boil), until Agar-Agar is completely dissolved. Add orange juice and pour into molds which have been rinsed with cold water. Refrigerate.

212. Vanilla Sauce*

3/4 cup milk
1/2 stick of vanilla beans
1 tbsp. sugar or fruit concentrate
1/4 tsp. cornstarch
1 egg
6 tbsp. cream if desired

Prepare vanilla creme, recipe No. 204. Beat cream until stiff and fold in.

213. Almond Milk Sauce*

1-1/2 cups milk
2 oz. almonds, peeled, ground
1-1/2 oz. honey
1 tbsp. cornstarch
2 tbsp. water

Bring to boil milk, almonds, honey. Mix cornstarch with cold water and stir into boiling milk. Blend this sauce well.

214. Rose Hip Sauce

2-1/2 oz. rose hip puree or rose hip paste
3/4 cup water or grape juice
2-1/2 oz. raw sugar or fruit concentrate
A few drops of lemon juice

Bring to a boil rose hip puree, water and sugar. Add lemon juice last.

215. Red Wine Sauce

3/4 cup water
lemon or orange peel
1 cinnamon stick
1 clove
2-2-1/2 oz. sugar or fruit concentrate
3/4 cup red grape juice
3/4 oz. almonds

Mix together water, peel, cinnamon, clove, and sugar. Boil a few minutes. Strain. Add grape juice and heat; do not boil. Peel almonds; cut into slivers and add.

216. Punch (non-alcoholic)

1-1/2 cups water
1-1/2 cups cider
1-1/2 cups red grape juice
1 slice of lemon
1/4 cinnamon stick
1 clove
4 tbsp. raw cane sugar
1 tbsp. lemon juice
3 tbsp. fruit syrup

Boil water with spices and lemon for 5 minutes; strain and add cider and grape juice. Heat again, add lemon juice, sugar, and syrup, and serve very hot.

217. Semolina Molds*

5-1/2 oz. semolina
3 pts. milk
1 pinch of salt
2-3 tbsp. raw sugar or fruit concentrate
1 egg, beaten
1 lemon peel, grated
1-1/2 oz. almonds, peeled and ground
1 oz. raisins
Raspberry syrup

Combine semolina and boiling milk, salt, and cook, adding sugar at the last. Add egg to farina; then lemon peel, almonds, and raisins. Rinse mold with cold water and fill with semolina mixture. Serve with raspberry syrup.

218. Red Grits

3 cups currant, raspberry or strawberry juice
1-1/8 cups red grape juice or water
2-1/2 oz. semolina
1 tbsp. cornstarch

Mix juices and bring to a boil. Stir in semolina and boil for 10 minutes. Mix cornstarch with a little cold water and add to the mixture. Rinse pudding mold with cold water and fill with mixture. Refrigerate.

Serve with vanilla sauce, recipe No. 212*, or almond milk, recipe No. 44, 45, 213.

219. Cottage Cheese Soufflé

1-1/3 oz. butter
4 tbsp. flour
1-1/8 cups milk, hot
1 lb. cottage cheese
2 eggs
2-1/2 oz. raw sugar

1-1/3 oz. raisins
Lemon peel, grated
4 tbsp. cream

Melt butter, add flour, and heat. Add milk and cook for a few minutes. Mix in cheese and eggs, sweetener, raisins and peel, and cream. Fill soufflé dish with the mixture and bake in the oven for 30-40 minutes.

V. Menus

Strict Diet Menu Plan for One Week

First Day

Breakfast: 1. Almond milk Muesli (sesame puree if desired).
2. Wholewheat bread or whole grain bread.
3. Nut puree.
4. Fruit (select from): Oranges, pears, apples, cherries, sour cherries, prunes, plums, watermelon, melon, tangerines, currants (red and black), bananas, dried figs, grapes.
5. Nuts: Almonds, hazelnuts, pecans, walnuts.
6. Tea: Herb tea, raw sugar.

Lunch: 1. Fruit: Choose from list given above.
2. Raw vegetables: Cauliflower, tomatoes, lettuce.
3. Cooked dishes: Beans, baked potatoes with caraway seeds.

Dinner: Same as breakfast, with the addition of spelt soup (recipe No. 64).

Second Day

Breakfast: The same every day.

Lunch: 1. Fruit: Choose from list given above.
2. Raw vegetables: Kohlrabi, lettuce.
3. Cooked dishes: Vegetable bouillon (made from onions, leek, green cabbage, potato peels, sorrel).
4. Cauliflower.
5. Parsley potatoes.

Dinner: Same as breakfast, with the addition of cooked cereal with grapes.

Third Day

Breakfast: As above.

Lunch: 1. Fruit: Choose from list given above.
2. Raw vegetables: Turnips, cucumbers, lettuce.
3. Cooked dishes: Green peas, steamed, in rice mold.
4. Fruit jelly, prepared with Agar-Agar.

Dinner: As above, with addition of thick potato soup.

Fourth Day

Breakfast: As above.

Lunch: 1. Fruit: Choose from list given above.
2. Raw vegetables: carrots, spinach, watercress.
3. Cooked dishes: Barley soup, steamed kohlrabi, potatoes with tomatoes.

Dinner: 1. Fruit and nuts.
            2. Crushed grain Muesli.
            3. Soaked dried prunes.

Fifth Day

Breakfast: As above.

Lunch: 1. Fruit: Choose from list.
            2. Raw vegetables: Beets, chicory, iceberg or Boston lettuce.
            3. Cooked dishes: lettuce, sautéed, stewed potatoes.
            4. Stuffed apples (with raisins and nuts).

Dinner: Same as breakfast.

Sixth Day

Breakfast: As above.

Lunch: 1. Fruit: Choose from list.
            2. Raw vegetables: Celery, Brussels sprouts, escarole.
            3. Cooked dishes: Brown wheat soup, cauliflower, steamed polenta.

Dinner: As above.

Seventh Day

Breakfast: As above.
Lunch: 1. Raw vegetables: Viper's grass, Romaine lettuce, Boston lettuce.
            2. Fruit: Choose from list.
            3. Cooked dishes: Brussels sprouts, steamed, Japanese whole grain rice.

4. Banana dessert.

Dinner: As above.

Mild Diet Menu Plan for One Week

First Day

Fruit, dried fruit.
Raw vegetables: carrots, endives, Boston lettuce.
Vegetable broth with bread cubes.
Viper's grass with lemon and cream.
Potatoes with tomatoes.

Second Day

Fruit, dried fruit.
Raw vegetables: beets, cucumbers, watercress.
Tomatoes filled with rice.
Lemon whip.

Third Day

Fruit.
Raw vegetables: celery, tomatoes, escarole.
Semolina soup.
Chopped cabbage.
Potatoes with caraway seeds.

Fourth Day

Fruit.
Raw vegetables: viper's grass, spinach, endives.
Polenta.
Apple Whip (without sugar).

Fifth Day

Fruit.
Raw vegetables: white radish, zucchini, Boston
   lettuce.
Vegetable soup.
Swiss chard in sauce.
Lyonnaise potatoes.

Sixth Day

Fruit.
Raw vegetables: cauliflower, watercress, Boston
   lettuce.
Chervil soup.
Spinach noodles with tomato sauce and cheese.

Seventh Day

Fruit.
Raw vegetables: raw stuffed tomatoes with celery
   salad and Boston lettuce.
Steamed squash with a little lemon juice.
Potato puree with tomatoes sprinkled with dry
   powdered herbs.
Almond pudding with raspberry syrup.

Breakfast: Bircher Muesli or fruit or fruit juice.
            Bread.
            Butter or nut puree
            Rose hip tea or herb tea.
            Nuts, grated or whole.

Supper: Bircher Muesli or
          Fruit or fruit salad or 1/2 grapefruit.
          Soup, bread, cheese or

Baked potatoes with cottage cheese, herbs and
   green salad, or
Sandwiches and green salad, etc.

See also *Eating Your Way to Health* by the Bircher-Benner Staff. Published by Penguin Books, Baltimore, Maryland: 1972.

An extended weekly diet plan should consist of:
   1 day—strict diet.
   1 day—raw vegetable diet with vegetable bouillon and
      baked potatoes.
   5 days—expanded lacto-vegetarian diet.

Any alcohol, sugar, coffee, tea, nicotine, and meat should be avoided for at least one year and should, thereafter, only be taken occasionally.